BLUNDERS IN THE GYM

Fitness Mistakes to Avoid for Physique Perfection

By Marshall A. Nash

i

Legal Notice and Disclaimer:

This publication is designed to provide competent and reliable information regarding the subject matter covered. However, it was written for informational and entertainment purposes only. It is sold with the understanding that the author and publisher are not engaged in professional advice, but rather the author is merely providing opinions and beliefs based on personal experiences and first-hand knowledge as a personal fitness trainer. It is the author's belief that the information provided is accurate, but the author and publisher specifically disclaim any liability that may be incurred from the use or application of the contents of this book. Fitness results are not guaranteed and are a result of an individual's personal efforts, knowledge, state of health, and other factors. Always seek the advice of your physician before beginning any exercise or nutritional plan.

Cover art by: Christoper Godsoe

Edited by: Nathan Chamberlain, Harmony L Williams, and Marshall Nash

Interior design by: Marshall Nash

Third Edition: January 2018

Library of Congress Control Number: 2016916133

CreateSpace Independent Publishing Platform, North Charleston, SC

ISBN-13: 978-1539009351

Printed in the United States of America

For Kenzie and Mikie

Acknowledgements:

Without the support and encouragement of my many friends and family, this book would not have been possible. I would like to thank my parents, Patty and Scott Chamberlain. My siblings Nathan Chamberlain and Michelle Poulin, my two best of friends Jared Sullivan, a.k.a Riff Johnson, my business partner and real-life local legend rock star; and Will Trogdon, my lifelong ranting and raving buddy whose lasting friendship have spawned countless interesting conversations. Special thanks to my brother and author Nate, aka Naters, for help with the editing process, and for being my inspiration to becoming a writer. A special thank you is also owed to my friend Harmony L Williams for a tremendous help with editing as well. I also want to give a special thanks to inspiring author Chris Godsoe for assistance with the cover design. I also need to thank all my workout partners I've had through the years because without your support and accountability I may never have achieved the kind of success I've had in the gym.

My very first workout partner was my childhood friend Rob Gerry. Countless hours were spent with the weights in my basement trying to get them veins to pop out and my muscles to bulge. My high school workout partners; my cousin Jacob Vanadestine who provided me with intense competition that propelled my results to the greatest of heights; and Josh Thomas whose strength I never could match, but motivated me to push that much harder each workout. My adult workout partners; Riff Johnson, who got me serious about weight lifting again after much time in hiatus, and who was pivotal in providing me the motivation to become an expert in this field and pursue my personal training certification. And finally my current workout partner, my cousin Jennifer Brawn. Jenn has inspired me to appreciate home-based workouts and cardio much more than I ever have, and whose discipline with diet has truly inspired me. I also need to give an acknowledgment to my fitness support group, the best and most fun support group in existence. This group consists of Will Trogdon, Nicole Trogdon, James Cowan, and myself. The competitive nature and banter in this group has brought me to the highest level of motivation, and has taught me the importance of a support network and how truly fun working in a group can be.

Contents

Introduction: *Let's Hit the Gym!*

The first time I ever touched a dumbbell I was seven years old. My stepdad had just moved in along with his pile of weights that made their way to our cellar. I was clueless about what to do with those little pieces of iron and cement-filled pieces of equipment. I started out by throwing those things around in dramatic fashion, hoping that somehow I would transform my little body into the likes of my childhood heroes of Arnold Schwarzenegger, Van Damme, Mark Wahlberg, and others. Since then, twenty-eight years later and countless gym memberships later, I've learned from every possible mistake a gym rat or bunny could make. I've personally witnessed time and time again people making the same blunders in the gym that are killing their chance of success.

I studied and studied what it took to get buff and ripped like my heroes. I even went out and earned a personal trainer certification, which mainly confirmed what I had already learned on my own, but I wanted the credibility. Earning my personal training certification also meant that I could help other people reach their goals. Helping others achieve their goals is something that I love to do. Fitness has always been my number one passion, and having gained all of this knowledge and experience over the years has prompted me to write this book so that I can share what I have learned with you.

My mission in writing this book is to reach as many people as I possibly can, to teach them what not to do and what has worked for me in the gym. If I can prevent people from repeating the same mistakes that myself and so many others do every day in the gym, then I will have accomplished my mission. This book is designed not just to show you the flaws being made in the gym, but it will also give you insight on what you should be doing as well. It has been written for everyone who has ever asked the questions "What am I doing wrong? Why am I not getting results? What do I need to be doing?" It is my hope that after reading this book you will be well on your way to success in the gym and achieving the body of your dreams! That's what we all want right? Who wouldn't want that? After you read this book, you'll be able to see these mistakes in action in almost any gym. Tell them they need this book!

Most people that go to the gym legitimately do not know what they need to do to achieve their goals, and as a result they make most, if not all of the mistakes that I will point out. They get frustrated with all of the effort, and the lack of results cause most people to quit. I want to change all that. With a little knowledge, this can all be turned around. I want every single individual who goes to the gym with a goal in mind to be informed well enough to know what it's going to take to get to where they want to be. This goal may be a lofty one, but I believe anything is possible. Once you've read this book you'll be very well informed, and you will be well ahead of the game. Good luck in the quest for your perfect body!

Chapter One: *Stop Talking!*

Lesson 1: Limit socialization/distractions.

One of the most common mistakes I have regularly witnessed at the gym is socializing to the point that your workout isn't much work at all. I've been very guilty of this common mistake myself. Surprisingly, out of all the technical mistakes that people make in the gym, this one can be one of the hardest to overcome. The reason being is we are social creatures. Socializing is typical behavior, and to shy away from that in a setting where talking with others can easily be done is often a bit challenging. However, what happens in many cases is socializing becomes a huge distraction from performing a good quality workout. Often what happens when you end up talking to your fellow gym rat, or the person on the bench you happen to be sharing with, is that the tempo of your workout slows way down, and you end up taking too long of breaks. Losing focus like this will absolutely affect the quality of your workout, and the quality of your workout is one of the biggest aspects of what will lead you to success, or in the absence of quality workouts, dismal to no results at all.

Working out for results is serious work, and requires your utmost attention. That is why the word "work" is included in the term "working out." Now I'm not saying you have to go to the gym and be a total social outcast and not say a word, or completely ignore people, but try to avoid getting into a lengthy conversation during the workout. Of course, talking before or after the workout would be perfectly fine. This blunder has been tough for me to avoid in the past, and I admit even to this day. If someone tries talking to me while I'm in the middle of a set, I try to give a nod until my set is over and then give the shortest possible response without coming across as rude. Unless I'm with a gym partner, I try to avoid starting a conversation with strangers in the gym, except of course if there's a purpose to speaking, such as asking if I can use that bench they're sitting on, etc. If I'm with a partner, naturally conversation will be part of the workout, but you can do so in a manner where you are only talking when you can take a quick breath. The primary focus needs to be on the workout, and the bulk of any conversation with a partner should be words of encouragement.

Another distraction you will find in almost any gym is television. The only time you should pay any significant attention to a TV hanging on the wall is when you're on the treadmill, or some stationary cardio machine that is placed right in front of any of the TVs. Of course, this is perfectly fine, and it can be a good distraction from the boredom that is often associated with doing cardio on a machine. However, if you're doing anything but working out in front of the TV, don't pay any attention to it. If you allow yourself to be distracted by a TV. the same way you can be with socializing, then you're going to have the same result: a lackluster workout that produces little, if any, results.

Instead of succumbing to distractions like these, this is what I strive to achieve in any given workout: one-hundred percent focus entirely on the work at hand. When you give your full attention to the moment you are in and what you are trying to accomplish, you will naturally do a better job. Remember this always: high-quality workouts over time equal high-quality results. In fact, part of the reason why working out is considered to be a good stress reliever is because when you are focusing all of your attention on the workout, you are not giving any attention to any of the stressors in your life. You're not worried about your job, relationships, money, or any of the other millions of stressors that bear down on us in everyday life. It gives your brain a break, and we all know it's good for the body, and I believe it's good for the soul.

Think of the mind-body connection. Let's say for example you're doing a bicep curl. If you focus completely and intently on the movement and the muscles involved in that movement, you strengthen that connection.[1] A strong mind-body connection is what I believe gives some athletes the advantage of "natural" skill that the majority of us simply don't have.[2] Using their skills over and over again turns on the auto perform button in their bodies and their natural talent takes over. That's my belief, in any case. It is also my belief that you can exercise this connection with intense focus and become much better at working out than those around you in the gym who are talking about the game last night, politics, or the date they had recently.

Ideally, having no distractions are what could produce the best results, but we live in an imperfect world. My advice to you is to do your best to limit any distractions that can hinder your performance to the best of your ability. Your cell phone can be a distraction. Turn it off, if that's feasible. Your iPod can even be a distraction. When you're busy trying to shuffle through to get to that one song, you are not working your body. Anything that distracts you from this purpose can be limited, or removed.

Chapter One Summary:

- **Avoid all distractions. Limit socialization.**

- **Pay no attention to televisions in the gym, unless you're using a stationary cardio machine.**

- **Avoid fiddling with your iPod.**

- **Turn off your cell phone if possible.**

- **Strengthen the mind-body connection with intense focus on the work at hand.**

Chapter Two: *Did He Really Just Do That?!*

Lesson 2: Keep proper form and do appropriate exercises.

We've all seen it. That one guy, or girl, who performs the craziest and most bizarre moves in the gym. Watching someone execute these insane moves can't help but make you wonder how that person doesn't have a broken neck, or a broken something! If you were to do a simple search on YouTube, you're guaranteed to find someone doing some odd looking moves that you've never seen before that looks ridiculous. For example, I've seen a guy put a cable behind his head, and do "head lifts" with a stack of weights. What this man was trying to accomplish is still a mystery to me. Was he trying to build a huge neck? Not only was this move extremely dangerous, I doubt it produced any positive results. In fact, he probably had a very sore neck the next day.

When it comes to doing appropriate exercises, and moving your body, a little common sense will go a long way. If it is a strange or awkward feeling movement, it probably isn't something you should be doing. If it looks weird, you probably shouldn't be doing it. If it causes pain or discomfort, you absolutely should not do it. Basic exercises are definitely appropriate to achieve results. You don't need to reinvent the fitness wheel to achieve real and lasting results. Now, doing something different and learning different kinds of moves is perfectly fine, as long as it is not causing any harm and produces some results.

Doing appropriate exercises that are safe is paramount to your success in the gym. The number one rule of the gym is safety. For one, it sucks, and sucks bad, to get an injury that will keep you out of the gym for any amount of time. That will kill your time and efforts that you've already put into the gym to get the results you're seeking. I know this first-hand all too well. I've seriously injured my lower back three separate times, and one of those times I could barely get out of bed! I remember I had great momentum at the time; some serious results were starting to become noticeable, and all of a sudden one wrong move and my back was hurt so badly I was out of the gym for an entire month! It takes a lot of time, persistence, and patience to get any noticeable results in the gym. In just a short amount of time all of those results that you have worked so hard for can be lost. And when I say short; a month out of the gym can negate many months of effort and results. Keep this in mind when you are going through your workouts because trust me, you do not want to have the agonizing experience of achieving results, just to lose them due to an avoidable injury.

I remember I injured my Achilles heel terribly one time while playing tennis. I play and compete extremely hard, and sometimes the result of that is an injury. That was another awful impairment that kept me from doing any leg work that required the use of my foot. I blame part of that injury on not having proper foot gear. When necessary, having quality personal equipment is another thing you have to keep in mind when working out, especially when it comes to footwear if you're doing any running or footwork.[3] Proper footwear can certainly help you prevent injury, and the wrong ones can be the cause of it.[3] For example, if you're a runner, running shoes are the best kind to wear in that situation.[3] I suggest wearing comfortable clothing in the gym as well. You don't want to be wearing tight, restrictive clothing when your body needs to be free in movement. Now, with doing proper exercises and with safety in mind, it is crucial to keep the correct form on each and every exercise that you perform.[4]

Keeping proper form on exercises is important for a few reasons, including safety and performance.[5] As I said before, we always keep safety rule number one in the gym. The other main reason for the importance of proper form is how it relates to your performance. One of my goals when working out is to always strive for the perfect rep or the perfect form during any exercise, no matter what it is. Keeping strict proper forms accomplishes two things. It keeps you hyper-focused on the task at hand, and it will get you the best results you can get from the movement or exercise that you are performing.[5] Staying hyper-focused will certainly increase your chances of achieving the perfect body you seek while strengthening the mind-body connection.[1]

Keeping proper form also means doing each rep or movement in the fullest possible range of motion.[6] An example would be a simple pushup. Going all the way up and all the way down is one complete rep, anything else doesn't count unless you're doing a specialized move to increase athletic performance, or trying to improve on a "sticking point." What I mean by that is this: when doing a pushup there is a certain point where you have the least amount of mechanical leverage, which is about half way upward on the pushup.[8] Get on the floor and try one pushup right now and you'll understand what I'm explaining. When you hit the sticking point, you are at the section in the movement where it is the hardest.[9]

Pretty much any exercise has a sticking point. With that being said, unless you are trying to improve your strength at this particular point in the motion by holding your body at this point, or doing quick short reps up and down through this narrow point, always execute the move with a full range of motion. You will engage more muscle fiber by doing the entire range of motion than shortening your reps, therefore getting better results.[7] Chances are unless you are an athlete and have a strength coach, this isn't a normal activity you would need to be doing. You don't need to get to that advanced of a level to achieve seriously impressive results. Usually, this kind of training is designed to get you to be excellent at certain specific movements, not to get overall head-turning results. Another thing to keep in mind when it comes to proper form is your breathing.

A common mistake that I've seen many times is someone holding their breath, particularly when they are lifting a heavy weight. This typical gym blunder is dangerous and counterproductive. First of all, holding your breath is going to raise your heart rate and blood pressure.[10] It puts undue stress on your body, and I strongly advise against it. Your body naturally requires more oxygen when you are working out, so remember to breathe. I also need to point out that there is a proper way to breathe when you work out. You breathe out during the concentric movement of an exercise, and you breathe in on the eccentric movement.[11] To explain what this means, consider a bicep curl. The concentric movement is when you are contracting the muscle.[12] In the case of a bicep curl, for example, it's when you lift the weight up towards your shoulder. The eccentric movement is when you are extending the muscle.[12] With a bicep curl it is the opposite of the concentric movement; when you bring the weight back down away from your shoulder. I will also point out that the eccentric movement is the most significant part of a repetition.[13] Controlling the weight on the way down in the bicep curl will strengthen and induce more growth than the concentric movement.[13]

I also want to point out that when it comes to your breathing, one good way to gauge the intensity of your cardio workout is if you can hold a conversation when you're working out, or you're breathing fast enough that talking becomes laborious. For example, if you are on a treadmill and

the person next to you is trying to have a
conversation, and you can easily talk back to the
person, you're not doing it right. You should be
working hard enough that you can't physically hold
a conversation. In another setting, such as just
walking to cool down or relax, or just doing a light
workout, it makes sense that you would not be
working so hard that you can't talk. Walking your
dog isn't so intense that you can't talk to someone
that may be walking with you. However, when you
are in the gym working your tail off trying to get that
perfect body, remember this rule.

Chapter Two Summary:

- **Safety is rule number one.**

- **Common sense goes a long ways. If it looks
  strange, feels awkward, or hurts, don't do
  it!**

- **Basic exercises WILL get you results!**

- Appropriate and safe exercises can help prevent deflating injuries.

- Having proper personal equipment, such as correct footwear can help prevent nagging injuries.

- Proper form is especially important for results and injury prevention.

- Using full-range of motion will yield the best results.

- Never hold your breath when lifting. Breathe in on eccentric movement, out on concentric.

- Eccentric movements are more important to strength than concentric movements.

- Cardio should be intense enough you can't easily carry on a conversation.

Chapter Three: *Fast "40"*

Lesson 3: Get in and get out.

There have been countless times when I have gone to the gym, done my workout, and there is at least one person that was there before I came to the gym and is still there when I'm leaving. After all the time I've spent before, during, and after my workout, that person will still be there slinging metal, pounding away on the treadmill, or doing some regimen even when I'm ready to hit the road. Better yet, they will just be walking around doing a little here and there during the entire time. A good rule of thumb is you should be able to work out no longer than one hour each session and still get amazing results. In fact, you don't even need to spend that much time working out if your intensity is at the right level. You can get results producing efficient workouts in thirty to forty minutes tops.[14] My workouts generally will last around forty minutes when I include a brief warm up and cool down, and I've gotten very noticeable results doing so.

When I was in high school, I was determined to get huge with weights and bodybuilding, but before I educated myself, you would find me slaving away in the gym for two hours at a time. I was certain this was the only way to get huge and to achieve the level of fitness I wanted to reach. That was entirely false! I did get incredible results back then in my prime testosterone producing days, but I could have gotten even better results if I had worked smarter, not harder and longer. Apparently, I'm not the only one that has made this mistake in the gym.

I've seen many other gym rats and bunnies spend hours upon hours in the gym just like I have in the past when it's not at all necessary. Let me ask you a question. If you could get the same, or even better results, in under an hour as you would in two hours a day at the gym, which would you rather do? Anything over an hour probably means you're training for the Olympics, professional bodybuilding is your career, or you're a professional athlete. If you are none of those you most likely have the same mindset that I had in high school. Or, your intensity is lackluster and you're just slowly going through the motions and spending your time at the gym ineffectively. They say that achieving one's fitness goals is a marathon, not a sprint. While that is true, each workout day should be a sprint. It is, in fact, a marathon of a collection of sprints. Quick, efficient, and sweat producing workouts are going to be much more productive than slowly going through the motions, or working out for so long that you risk overtraining, or boring yourself to death. Too much of anything is a bad thing, even when it comes to fitness.

Chapter Three Summary:

- **No more than one hour is needed at the gym at the right intensity level.**

- **Too much of anything is bad. Lengthy gym time can lead to boredom or overtraining.**

Chapter Four: *Sweat and Don't Repeat!*

Lesson 4: Mix it up, or you will go stale.

Working the same muscle groups every day, or doing the same workout routine over and over again, is like being the hamster on the wheel, worse actually. This blunder is yet another common mistake that I have seen too many times to count. You will not make progress working the same muscle groups every day; in fact, you will regress rather than make progress.[15] If you're working the same muscles every day, you are not giving your muscles a chance to repair themselves, and to get stronger and adapt to the load you are putting on them.[16] When you work out, especially when lifting weights, you are breaking down muscle fibers and causing tiny little micro-tears in the fibers.[15] When you rest those muscles, this is when strength changes and growth will occur.[16] The reason being is because when your body repairs its muscle tissue, it is trying to restore itself to a state of adaptation to the load you just previously placed on it.[16] When you work out the same muscles every day and don't give them a chance to heal, you will continue to break them down further and further until they become so fatigued that you can't even perform at the same level you did the day before.[16] This breaking down will continue until you give your body a chance to heal, or it breaks down to the point of utter exhaustion, and you just can't perform much at all.[16] Your body will begin to use muscle as fuel if you continue to pound away intensely on the same muscles every day.

If you're just doing light to moderate exercises, it would be ok to work the same or similar muscles every day.[17] An example of that would be most any light to moderate intensity cardio. It is ok to jog every day because you're not putting such a heavy load on the muscles being worked that you could only jog every other day.[17] Your muscles can heal in a shorter amount of time in between light jogging sessions as compared to doing something along the lines of intense weight training. On the other hand, if you are doing some high impact intense cardio, you may need more time in between workouts to heal up. It's when you workout with enough intensity that you cause the tiny muscle fiber tears, that you need to give your body ample rest in between the workouts that are working the same muscles. A good example of this is if you do weight lifting, and you worked your chest on Monday; don't work your chest again on Tuesday. Wait until Wednesday at the earliest.[16]

An obvious indication that you have worked your muscles to the point of microscopic tears is being sore the next day, and especially two days later. Soreness the day after a workout is called "delayed-onset muscle soreness".[18] You should give the muscles you just worked at least forty-eight hours of rest in between workouts. I'll point out that conditioned muscles tend to heal faster than someone who is out of shape, or hasn't worked out in a while.[18] However, being conditioned doesn't mean you don't follow the forty-eight-hour rule; it does, however, mean that you will be less and less sore the more you are conditioned and the more you do the same routine. The healing process is so important to getting your results. It's during this stage where the actual transformational changes occur in your body. Working out does the tearing down, and the healing builds the body to a stronger, better state.

There are a few exceptions to the rule of not working the same muscles every day. Cardio is a unique exception that I have previously pointed out. Technically, you can do cardio every day as long as you are not running a marathon on a daily basis. Cardio doesn't tear down your muscles the same way weights do. The primary function of cardio is to work the heart and lungs, and they can do an unbelievable amount of work if you condition them right. Although you can do cardio every day, in my opinion, I believe it is wise to give yourself at least one day a week for complete rest. You risk burning out if you don't give yourself a break at least once in a while. In regards to specific muscles, when it comes to your abs, calves, and forearm muscles, these can be worked every day.[19]

These muscles are naturally designed and conditioned to be able to withstand everyday loads on them, even heavy loads.[19] Your abs and core need to be worked every day, or you couldn't even do simple tasks such as walking.[19] Your core is involved in the movement of the human body much more than you might think. Your calves can take heavy loads; otherwise, there would be days you couldn't even walk. Considering the survival nature of our species, in ancient times this would have made us inferior, and that's just not how we are as a species. The same applies to your forearms. The human body is designed to be able to grab, pull, and pick up things on a daily basis.[19] Unless you are working these muscles at an extremely intense level, or those muscles are very sore the next day after working them, you can work them every day. Even with all this said you still want to give your body ample rest even for these body parts. The typical eight hours of sleep a night should suffice, but, if you're doing an excessively challenging workout program, even up to ten hours of sleep a night may be necessary.[20] However, even if you are resting your muscles appropriately, just like I suggested, you don't want to do the same routine for months on end.

There are a couple of reasons why you don't want to continue the same routine over and over again. For starters, it can get extremely boring. I've been a victim of gym boredom before. It can without a doubt kill your motivation. Having fun, as crazy as that may sound, is another important rule of the gym you should follow; not far behind safety. Yes, you can have a good time working out. Getting visible results after patiently waiting for it to happen with all your hard work can be exhilarating, and can feel like a natural high. Visualize where you want to be and know that the work you're putting in now will get you there over time. That's part of the fun. It can also be fun because after a while you can become very conditioned, which will undoubtedly make you feel really, really good. You'll enjoy a better quality of life just simply being in excellent shape. Working out can actually become addicting, and you will seek it out and want to do it. There's also a real thing called the "runner's high." You may have heard of this. What can start to happen after working out is endorphins are released in your brain.[21] These are the "feel good" natural chemicals that your brain produces just by simply working out.[21] Runners experience this a lot, and that is why some people actually get addicted to running. Some even to the point where they do it too much, and remember, too much of anything can turn something good into something bad. You can experience this with weight lifting as well. I know this from personal experience.

When I was in my weight lifting heydays back in my testosterone prime high school years, I would experience this from time to time. I remember there being times I would get giddy from feeling so incredibly good. Jokes were funnier, I smiled a lot more (sometimes to the point of looking foolish), and I just felt overwhelmingly happy at times. However, this high was temporary, and I suspect it is for anyone else experiencing it. It is a good, natural, healthy high though and I recommend it for anyone. With that being said, if you are doing the same routine over and over again, you may still be able to get an endorphin rush, but there is a good chance that it will get boring, and you'll get to the point of just not wanting to do it. The other reason for not doing the same routine over and over again is to avoid the ugly and hated word "plateau."

Your body can only adapt so much to the load you put on it. When you've maxed out the adaptation you can achieve, you have hit a plateau.[22] The quickest and easiest way to hit this wall is to simply do the same routine day in and day out, or month in and month out. However, the opposite is true when you mix things up once in a while. What I recommend to any of my personal training clients is not to do the same routine for more than six weeks at a time. At that point, you can start to get close to the "this is starting to get boring" stage, or plateauing. By mixing things up, you are doing what's called "muscle confusion". Your muscles can't fully max out adaptation if you're putting different loads on them periodically.[23]

Any good workout program, or good trainer, will not prescribe you a routine that does not change after a short time. In fact, some workout programs will change after the first month. The changes don't have to be drastic, and in most cases, the changes only need to be small to prevent a plateau or boredom. There are countless different exercises you can do for each muscle group that will work them out in various and sometimes interesting ways. The pushup, for example, is a pretty straightforward move, but there are dozens of variations of pushups that will work the same or similar muscles at different angles and in unique ways. It is the same with many exercises. If you don't have a personal trainer to mix things up for you, and you're not familiar with different exercises, doing a simple Google search will show you a multitude of different kinds of exercises and the muscles that they use.

Chapter Four Summary:

- **Working the same muscles every day can lead to regression, not progression.**

- Rest is an important ingredient to gym success. Healed muscles become stronger muscles.

- An exception to the rule: light exercises such as jogging can be performed daily.

- Cardio can be performed daily, but a good rule of thumb is to fully rest at least one day a week.

- Other exceptions to the rule: your abs, calves, and forearms are designed for daily use, even heavy use.

- Muscle soreness is an indication for needed rest since muscle soreness comes from the breakdown of muscle tissue.

- During the healing process is when actual body transformation occurs.

- Eight hours of sleep normally suffices. High-intensity workouts can call for up to ten hours of sleep if this is feasible.

- **Mix up your routine periodically to prevent boredom, and plateauing.**

- **Change, or mix up your routine at least every six weeks. This creates "muscle confusion," an important tactic to achieving results.**

- **Most exercises have multiple variations of the same movement. This can aid you in muscle confusion.**

- **Having fun is a real gym rule, right behind safety. Working out can become addicting from the feel-good endorphins, such as the "runners high."**

Chapter Five: *Mr. Perfect Where Did You Go?!*

Lesson 5: Being consistent is always a winner.

I believe that if everyone who ever wanted their perfect body to become a reality was one-hundred percent consistent in getting their workouts done day in and day out there would be a whole lot of ripped bodies walking the earth today. Being consistent with working out is an everyday struggle for a lot of people, and I'm no exception. Out of all the possible blunders to make, this one I have probably struggled the most within the past. However, the more consistent I've been, the more results I've always gotten, without exception. Consistency is one of the hardest obstacles to overcome in anyone's journey to earning the body of their dreams.

For anyone, there will be days where you just don't have the drive or desire to work out, but if you genuinely want to be the master of your body you have to push through that and do it nevertheless.

The good news is once you've completed your workout that you so dreaded to do, you'll feel so much better for getting it done. If you don't push through that wall, you may regret it and ask yourself why didn't I just do it? Or you may not feel like that at all, but instead months down the road you'll be kicking yourself for not sticking with your workout because you know you would be way ahead of the game if you had just done the workouts every time, no matter what.

Here's what can happen if you skip a workout here and there on the days you just can't get out of your own way and get it done. Chances are you may end up skipping more and more workouts and eventually, you stop altogether. Unfortunately, I've been very guilty of this. There have been many times where I have started a routine, done well for a while, then I'll miss a workout or two, then life gets in the way and instead of staying committed, I find myself straying from the gym or completely stopping my workouts altogether. Then what happens is I end up doing the very same thing I just mentioned; regretting the fact of not sticking with it because three months down the road from when I stopped, I knew I would be in much better shape, and maybe even totally ripped by then. You will be so glad if you avoid this mistake of not being consistent. It takes incredible strength in willpower to do it, but that's the beauty of the human spirit. I believe anyone is capable of overcoming hardship and obstacles and doing amazing things if you sincerely want something bad enough.

It absolutely won't be easy to avoid skipping any of your workouts. I'm not going to lie; it will be incredibly hard. There will undoubtedly be times when you feel that you just don't have the time. The timing will never be right for anyone embarking on a journey to greatness, no matter what the endeavor may be, or how big or small your goals and dreams are. You just have to do it there's no way around it. Set aside the time that you need. People always seem to find the time to do the things that they really want to. Even if you don't want to, you have to make the time to get your workouts in. A half hour is not that much time out of your day. Carve out a small slice of time for yourself during the day and you won't regret it down the road. You are worth that time for yourself. A better you is the reward, and being a goal achiever is always better than being a quitter. You will feel a whole lot better when you achieve your goals as opposed to giving up.

I'm willing to bet that even the most famous athletes and bodybuilders, such as the likes of Arnold Schwarzenegger, had days just like we all do where working out feels like the lowest of priorities, and they struggle to find the willpower, but they did it regardless. There simply is no room for excuses of any kind if you want that perfect body. You have to make it a priority. Think of your health. Your health has a direct impact on the quality of your life. Feeling good and looking good will only make your world a happier place. Being healthy and fit is the real benefit of staying consistent in the gym, looking good is just a bonus. Even if your number one motivator is to look good at the beach, doing your workouts can improve your health even if you're not thinking about it, so get it done. It makes things a bit easier if you can form a habit of working out. It typically takes about three weeks to develop a habit.[24] Once you've made it habitual to work out, it can seamlessly become part of your life, and you'll just do it without much thought. If you can accomplish this, the battle will tip in your favor.

Chapter Five Summary:

- **One of the biggest blunders you can make is being inconsistent with your workouts.**

- **Push yourself to get your workouts in, even when you feel the least motivated, you will always feel glad you did after the workout is complete.**

- **Being healthy and fit is the real benefit of staying consistent in the gym, looking good is just a bonus.**

- **It can take up to three weeks to develop a habit. If you can make working out habitual, you are on your way to victory.**

Chapter Six: *Arnold Wasn't Built in a Day*

Lesson 6: Avoid the temptation to overtrain. Be patient for results.

In reality, Arnold built his legendary physique over the course of many years, and by the force of sheer commitment, focus, and determination. These are all key elements to success in anything, with the gym being no exception. He did not develop his amazing body in a short period of time by any means. If that were possible, we would be seeing a lot more Arnolds walking the earth. His drive was unparalleled in the universe of bodybuilding, and with hard work and time, he achieved all of his goals that he set out to accomplish, even those not related to bodybuilding. Waiting to see results from your workouts can be an extremely painful process, especially if having patience is a personal challenge. Patience is something that I have struggled with my entire life. I'm most certainly not what someone would consider a patient man. I'm an instant gratification kind of person, a flaw that I continue to attempt to eradicate.

It's no secret that Arnold Schwarzenegger was one of my childhood heroes. I can honestly say watching his movies when I was a kid, was what inspired me to start lifting weights. I would train for hours on end trying to build mountains of muscle so that I could be like my hero. One thing I was unaware of back then in my younger years was the fact that you can overtrain, but I learned about it the hard way. As I've said before, too much of anything is bad, no matter what it is. Overtraining is a severe and real condition that you can put yourself into if you're not careful. I've already mentioned about the rule of not working the same muscle groups every day, but even if you follow that rule you can still overtrain if you overdo it.

If you are overtraining, you will start to lose in the gym. Your motivation will decline. You will start to feel extremely fatigued, and your performance will undoubtedly suffer. When you've reached the state of overtraining your body, you cannot recover fast enough in between workouts.[25] Your body's energy sources have been depleted, and if you continue to work out at an intense level, your body will start to break down until you've reached complete and utter exhaustion. You do not want to develop the condition of your body being overtrained. The only way to reverse the state of being overtrained is complete rest, and this process can take quite some time to completely undo, even months if it is bad enough.[25] Because you need complete rest, you obviously have to stop working out altogether and get as much rest as humanly possible to recover in the shortest amount of time. In the meantime though, you're not training, and this will set you back. This could equate to months' worth of hard work going right down the drain. Overtraining syndrome is one reason why rest is so important. Without proper rest, you increase your chances of suffering from this condition.[25]

Being overzealous can lead you down this dangerous path of overtraining. As painful as it is, you just have to patiently wait for the results to show up in the mirror. Everybody that's just starting out goes through this painful process, but once you start getting results, they can be more motivating than almost anything else. Seeing the fruit of your efforts will make you feel elated. It will make you want to keep working harder to see even more results. Results can become a healthy addiction; but remember, results take time, and there will be small subtle ones that you may not notice at first. Usually what happens is that people you don't see very often will notice the changes first. Since they don't see you every day, little things become more apparent. Others seeing these changes can be motivating because it validates that what you are doing is bearing fruit, rather than being fruitless. It can be extremely hard waiting for those results to come through, but trust me, in the end, they are very much worth it, and will help propel you forward.

Chapter Six Summary:

- **Overtraining is a real condition that proves too much of anything can be bad.**

- **Overtraining will lead to extreme fatigue, loss of motivation, and lackluster performance.**

- **Complete rest is the only way to reverse the condition of overtraining. This can take some time, even months in extreme cases.**

- **Since complete rest is required to correct an overtraining condition this can set you way back. Months of hard work can be erased very quickly.**

- **Results take time, be patient. Results are very motivating because you are seeing the fruit of your labor manifest itself. Achieving results can become a healthy addiction.**

Chapter Seven: *Slug Syndrome*

Lesson 7: Never lack intensity.

A lack of intensity is probably one of the biggest reasons why a lot of people never see any results with their workouts. There is a wall. It's called "your limitations". Everyone has them, but rarely do the people who don't see results ever come up against that wall and try to push through it. In order to move forward and see progress, you have to push against your limitations. There's no way around it, and there are no shortcuts. You can't become better at anything unless you actually attempt to do it better. Intensity is one of the key ingredients that are essential to getting the needed work done that will show up in the mirror down the road. A lot of times I see people just sort of going through the motions going from one exercise to the next, barely looking like they're doing anything at all. They hardly break a sweat. If the workout isn't hard, you're not doing it right. If it doesn't make you sweat, chances are you're not doing it right. And as I have said before, if you are doing cardio and you can hold a conversation with the same ease that it takes while sitting on the couch or going for a walk, it isn't hard enough.

Intensity is simply how hard the work is. If it's hard, that's a good thing. That's what you want. The ole cliché is true; if it were easy, everyone would do it. The harder it is the more meaningful the work becomes. Victory is so much sweeter when it is earned, and you can't obtain that perfect body you've been dreaming of without hard work and pushing through your limitations. Meet your limitations head-on; challenge them, beat them, and you will find your ability to soar to new heights. Go through the pain and struggle now and come out on the other side a better version of yourself. A lack of intensity will only hold you back, and the lack of results will only frustrate you, and when you're disappointed, your chance of failure or quitting increases. Work hard now; stick with it and I guarantee that you won't regret it. Quitting produces regret, and regret is one of the worse feelings in the world, at least in my opinion. If no one ever caused themselves any regret I believe it'd be a much happier world we live in.

Chapter Seven Summary:

- **A lack of intensity is perhaps the biggest blunder of them all, and the number one reason why some never see results from their workouts.**

- **In order to progress, you must push against your limitations. New limitations are only attained by pushing past old ones.**

- **If the workout isn't hard and doesn't make you break a sweat, you're not doing it right.**

- **Victory is much sweeter when it's earned. Earn it.**

Chapter Eight: *My Cousins Uncle Said So*

Lesson 8: Be wary of whom you take advice from.

There's always that one person who knows everything about everything. Besides the fact that this simply isn't possible, it's incredibly annoying. The gym is without a doubt one place you can be certain to run into someone like this. More times than not, you can count on this person to have all kinds of advice for you and how you're doing something wrong. I honestly don't believe these kinds of "experts" are purposely trying to sabotage your workouts, and in fact, most of them probably have good intentions, but sometimes it seems as if they like to hear themselves talk and to sound all-knowing and relevant. Take everything they say with a grain of salt, and keep in mind you can always do your own research to see if what they say is true if you feel like spending your time doing so.

Sometimes you may get good advice, but if you don't already have the knowledge yourself, it can be hard to tell. Unless someone has been trained and is a personal trainer or fitness expert of some caliber, you can't take what they say as gospel. Not only that but everyone's body will react differently to different stimuli, so what works for them doesn't always translate into guaranteed success for you.[26] I will touch on this later, but just as an example, some may notice they get better results working with machines than they do free weights. That's not to say you shouldn't incorporate them both into your workouts for different reasons, but I'll go into that later in the Tid Bits of Fit section of this book.

The point to remember is that some people just flat out don't know what the hell they're talking about. An excellent example of this was an encounter I had while I was doing my internship for my personal training certification. The trainer I was working with had an older client doing what she called "negative pull-ups." Basically what was happening is the client wasn't at a strength level at the time to do a full pull-up. What the trainer was having this individual do was stand on a chair while holding the bar (he was at the top of the position of a pull-up), and then he would slowly lower himself to the ground with his feet off the chair. Lowering himself down was the negative move in the pull-up, hence the term negative pullups. He would do this ten times for three sets. At one point the trainer had to go to the bathroom and left me to guide the client. As soon as this took place a guy came up to me and told me that having this customer do negative pullups won't help him one bit, he told me you couldn't build any muscle or strength that way. Not looking to get into an argument with a complete stranger, especially since I was just an intern at the time, I simply thanked him and continued the workout as we were doing regardless.

First off, this stranger was completely wrong and had no idea what he was talking about. The client was trying to build up to being able to do one full pull-up without the assistance of the chair. Having him attempt a regular pull-up at this point would have been moot; he wouldn't even have been able to do one rep. Having him do negative pullups would increase the strength in the muscles used in the exercise, and as I've pointed out earlier, the negative motion (eccentric) of any exercise is more important than the positive (concentric) movement in terms of building strength and muscle growth.[27] So this stranger had no idea what he was talking about.

The way I handled it is how I would suggest anyone should deal with advice from strangers, especially when they don't know the truth about what they are saying. Just simply thank them and move on. It isn't worth getting into a debate or an argument over, and will waste your time and distract you from your workout. I remember when the trainer returned I told her the story of what had just happened. She chuckled and said "Well, we know that's false." You will always get people that will give you false information like that thinking that it's sound advice. I've gotten advice like this in the past a few times.

My advice would be to only trust the words from a professional, such as a personal trainer like myself, and trust your own instinct. If something doesn't seem right or sounds phony, it likely is. Don't be surprised if you experience something similar to what I have more than once when someone tries to tell you that you're not doing it right, or tell you what you should be doing. Keep in mind some people genuinely want to help, but some just like to sound intelligent. Good gym Samaritans may have good intentions, but if you take their advice as golden, then you risk being led astray.

Chapter Eight Summary:

- **There are always "experts" who will try to give you advice. Take what they say with a grain of salt.**

- **Everyone's body reacts differently to different kinds of stimuli (weight training, cardio, etc.)**

- **Avoid getting into arguments with know it all's; simply say thanks for the advice and move on. It's not worth the distraction and** energy to engage with these kind of "good Samaritan gym patrons."

- Only trust the words from professionals, such as personal trainers like myself, and trust your own instinct. If something doesn't seem right or phony, it likely is.

Chapter Nine: *I Like Ice Cream!*

Lesson 9: Always make diet priority number one.

Even though your diet is not a direct gym blunder, one cannot have a fitness book without the discussion of diet, and the title of this topic absolutely rings true for me. Ice cream is by far my favorite food. It has been since I was a little pipsqueak. Anyone who knows me knows this to be true. Sweets have always been my Achilles heel, my kryptonite you could say. I've struggled most of my life with diet and being addicted to food, and especially sugar. As of this writing, my diet is looking pretty good, though, and the better my diet has been, the better my results have always been as well.

When it comes to how you look, and contrary to what some may believe, diet actually trumps your workouts, and is extremely critical to your success in the gym and your overall health. I can't stress enough how important one's diet truly is. You see, diet gives you a base to work with; you could call diet the hammer. The workouts are the chisel that works out the rough edges of the underlying masterpiece. Combining a strong, disciplined diet with good consistent quality workouts is very powerful in aiding you with achieving that stunning body of your dreams. I believe when it comes to diet and exercise, and the effect it has on your appearance is 80/20. Eighty percent is diet, twenty percent is exercise, so you need to make diet priority number one.[28] Here are some of the most common diet mistakes I've seen before, and some tips on the right things to do when it comes to your diet.

It's easy to make the mistake of thinking you can eat whatever you want and still get results in the gym; especially when you are young and your metabolism is higher than your adulthood years. This is something I thought to be true for years. In fact, up until a few years ago, I believed that since I worked out so hard whatever I ate would just turn to muscle. Man was I clueless. I truly thought I could eat whatever I wanted, and it didn't matter. I was uneducated on this issue, and nothing could be farther from the truth. You can ruin all the hard work you put into a workout with one poor food choice. The slice of cheesecake that takes less than five minutes to scarf down will ruin that hard hour-long workout that you just put in at the gym.

When I was younger, it was incredibly easy to build muscle and keep fat off, even without a perfect diet. My metabolism was on turbo back then. All of this started to change as I got older, and my waistline started creeping outwards. Around the age of 33 was when I first began to notice that food seemed to pack on weight at a much quicker rate than before. Even if you are young, and it's not hard to keep fat off, this line of thinking will prevent you from reaching your body's full potential. How is that so? Food is the fuel for your workouts; the better the fuel, the better the workouts. The better the workouts you perform, the better the results. In my opinion, food can also be your medicine. It can make you feel good, or it can be your poison and make you feel awful. It can affect your mood, your energy level, and most definitely will affect your overall health. Eating right should be done at any age, and you certainly will notice the effects of bad eating over time with age. Another mistake people make with their diet is that they simply have poor eating habits.

It's not just what you eat, although that's imperative, but how much you eat and when you eat plays a factor as well. Eating too much of anything, even what is considered healthy food, can make you fat. Overeating will kill your chances of success in the gym. Overeating is something I've certainly struggled with in the past. It seems the older I got, the more I loved food, but I had to get my bad habit of overeating under control if I ever wanted to get real lasting results in the gym. In my view, it's better to eat five small meals a day rather than three big ones like the standard American diet.[29] Have your breakfast, a mid-morning snack, lunch, a mid-afternoon snack, and then dinner.

Eating every few hours will help keep your blood sugar stable, which is important when it comes to fat and weight control.[30] Keeping your blood sugar level stable will also help you keep a good steady level of energy as well.[30] As long as you're not consuming vast amounts of sugar, you won't experience the kind of sugar spike and crash that is commonly associated with a diet high in sugar, and eating irregularly.[30] When your blood sugar spikes, your body has to get the level back down as quickly as possible, which causes fat storage and the infamous crash that I'm sure we've all experienced at one point in our lives.[30] Keeping your blood sugar stable will also help with your mood.[30] A better mood usually will go hand in hand with better motivation; this all factors into the quality of your workouts.

One way to keep your blood sugar relatively even is to eat slower digesting foods.[30] One way to you can accomplish this is to eat a protein with every meal, including your snacks throughout the day.[30,32] Having an apple? Ok, eat some peanut butter with it. Protein digests slower than carbs and won't cause your blood sugar to increase as quickly as eating a simple carb. The hierarchy of the ease of digestion is as follows: simple carbs like sugar digest the quickest, complex carbs like fruits and vegetables would be next on the list, then proteins, fats, and then fiber.[31] It's my belief that if you combine a slower digesting food with a faster one, it could have the effect of slowing the quick - digestible food down, aiding in a slower steady increase in blood sugar. That's why I think it is a good idea to eat a protein with every meal, and it's the advice I received from one of the trainers at the gym where I completed my personal training internship. Also, I will point out for those who wish to put on muscle, I recommend eating at least one gram of protein per pound of body weight.[33] You need the extra protein to help build muscle. On the flip side of that coin, if you are trying to lose weight you shouldn't need to eat more than half the number of grams of protein per pound of body weight.[34] Another useful tip for those looking to lose weight that I see people mistakenly do a lot is drinking fruit juice.

Don't be deceived by the word "fruit". Juice is a power punch of sugar. I wouldn't consider it as bad for you as something like soda because juice does have some nutritional value to it, but if you drink a glass of juice, I hope you are not diabetic. It can cause the same kind of sugar high or spike as anything else that's loaded with sugar, and we all know this is not conducive to losing weight. Part of the problem with fruit juice is it doesn't have the same fiber content as a whole piece of fruit, and it's the equivalent of several pieces of fruit, hence the overload of sugar content.[35] Instead of drinking a glass of apple juice, eat an apple. Instead of drinking orange juice, eat an orange. You get the point. You'll be getting far less sugar, and you'll also be getting all the fiber that comes along with the whole piece of fruit, which will aid in slowing down the absorption of the sugar so that you don't get the sugar high that you would with drinking a glass of juice. Sugar is much worse than fat.[36]

Fat, especially healthy fat from things like nuts or fish, eaten in the right quantities will not make you fat; sugar, on the other hand, can grow that waistline quicker than any other food.[36] Also, I will point out that it's better to eat whole foods in general, and not processed garbage foods you see everywhere at the grocery store.[37] Whenever possible, it's better to eat food in its most natural state. For example, eating veggies raw rather than cooked is better for you. You will get the most nutrients out of the veggies that way. If you are to cook veggies (it's better to steam them), you'll retain more nutrients that way as opposed to boiling them, which will cause nutrients to leach out of the food and into the water.[38] Obviously, some foods require cooking, such as meat for example, but whenever possible, try to eat your vegetables raw. I also want to point out that the timing of when you eat plays a factor too.

I recommend not eating anything at least three hours before you go to bed at night. Eating at nighttime has always been a struggle for me as it seems as though I am always more hungry later in the evening. I have some theories as to why that is, but I can't for sure pinpoint where that comes from. The problem with eating too close to bedtime is that the food will likely be stored as fat that you will need to burn off later.[39] A lot of people eat supper and go to sleep shortly after. I've seen that a lot. If you're one of them, stop doing that, because it's one of the easiest ways to pack on some pounds and it can also disturb your sleep. I will say the same thing about working out too close to bedtime. I wouldn't recommend working out within at least three hours of going to bed. Working out too close to bedtime can disturb your sleep as well since you'll be stimulated, and it can take hours for your body to return to a more relaxed state after working out.[39]

Some might think that if I work out really hard I'll be tired and want to go to bed, but it usually has the opposite effect. You want to reap all the possible benefits you can from your workouts, with one being calorie burning. You don't burn as many calories in your sleep, and since your metabolism jacks up after a workout out you can burn extra calories for hours after working out.[40] Being awake will naturally help you take advantage of this benefit.

Another thing is to not eat too fast and take your time eating. Do not over indulge and exercise good portion control. It takes roughly twenty minutes for your brain to signal that you are full, so it is important to take your time eating.[41] Eat slowly and enjoy your food; there's nothing wrong with enjoying what you're eating, but just don't overdo it. The types of food, of course, play a role in your success for ultimate fitness as well.

I highly recommend limiting simple carbs, such as white bread or anything considered "junk food" in your diet, and instead focus on complex carbs, such as what you would get from eating fruits and vegetables.[42] In fact, I would recommend that the bulk of your diet be somewhere in the vicinity of at least fifty percent of your daily food intake be plant-based foods like vegetables and fruits. Make vegetables the number one food you eat, followed by fruit, proteins, fats, and then simple carbs. I suggest making sugary sweets or junk food dead last in the list of priority foods, or simply don't eat that awful food at all. With this being said, I have to give some attention to the "cheat meal."

I don't think having a cheat meal once in a while, maybe once a week, is a terrible idea, but at the same time your body never actually requires you to put junk in it. It's my belief that the purpose of the cheat meal is entirely psychological. Not giving yourself a break once in a while from eating superbly well and indulging in yummy bad food now and again, can put a lot of pressure on your motivation and stress level. For me, it's like a release from tension. I can't really call it a reward because it doesn't benefit your body at all as you're not putting quality fuel in it, but giving in once in a while could prevent you caving into the high pressure of being perfect with your diet and breaking down and binge eating. I've personally experienced this.

It's my opinion that in a worst case scenario if you are perfect eighty-percent of the time with your diet, then you are doing well enough that some serious changes can happen to your body. And cutting anything bad out of your diet cold turkey can make your cravings go through the roof, at least that's been my experience, and in my opinion, that's a common diet mistake unless you have superhuman willpower. It's better to weed the bad stuff out, indulge only once in a great while, and slowly retrain your taste buds into liking more healthy foods. Weeding the junk out is the best way to kick a bad diet habit in my view. If you are addicted to sugar, give your taste buds a good amount of time, possibly months to completely rid your brain and body of that addiction. If you are craving sweet stuff, reach for some fruit. Surprisingly, one thing that can affect your appetite is your workouts.

Whether you are doing strength training or doing some cardio, they each will have a different effect on your appetite. From what I've experienced and what others have told me, doing strength training, especially weight lifting, increases appetite.[43] This makes sense considering that in order for your body to adapt to the weights it has to add muscle; your body cannot create muscle without a stimulus (weight training, strength training, etc.), and food. However, the opposite can occur when you do cardio. Cardio tends to suppress appetite.[43] Since cardio works your heart and lungs more so than weightlifting, the effect isn't for your body to build as much muscle as weight lifting, so therefore your appetite does not need to increase. Another important part of your diet that can't be overlooked is your fluid intake.

Being hydrated is crucial to your success in the gym and your overall health. Drinking enough water can make the difference between a high-quality workout and one that you struggle to get through. My recommendation is to ignore the typical recommended eight 8-ounce glasses a day. Throw that right out the window. There is no one size fits all when it comes to hydration. I base my recommendations on what I've discovered through my own research; how much an individual should drink depends on three factors; it depends on your weight, activity level, and what kind of climate you live in.[44] The amount you should drink is half to one ounce of water per pound of weight.[44] For example, if you weigh 200 pounds, you should drink between 100-200 ounces a day. If you're highly active and live in a hot climate, you should drink closer to the 200 mark.[44] If you're relatively sedentary and live in a cold area, you don't need as much water and would be okay being towards the lower end.[44] Keeping yourself hydrated will keep your metabolism operating at peak efficiency, and help with digestion as well.[44] On the other hand, if you are dehydrated it can affect your performance in the gym because virtually every chemical reaction in your body requires water to function properly.[45] Naturally, that means if you're not getting enough fluids you won't be able to train as hard in the gym. And now I have to turn your attention to the almighty calorie. One cannot talk about diet without talking about calories.

I cringe when I hear the term "a calorie is a calorie is a calorie!" Whoever coined this term needs a pie to the face; this statement is so untrue and damaging in my opinion. It's almost like saying just eat whatever you want, just make sure you eat less and move more. For your health's sake do not heed this moronic advice. When it comes to weight loss, I will admit that fewer calories in than out will naturally induce weight loss. Barring any medical condition inhibiting your ability to lose weight I will not argue that point that fewer calories in than out will cause weight loss, but to imply all calories are equal is outright ludicrous. I seriously hope that there are not many dietitians that still use this term, or even remotely agree with it. The term really should be better quality calories, better healthy body.

What you put in your body matters, and food isn't just a number. Otherwise, calories would be the only things that matter when it comes to consuming food. If you were to eat the same amount of calories that is contained in a Snickers bar or the same amount of calories by eating lettuce, I think you will find that you'll feel a whole lot better with the obviously wiser choice of salad. With the salad, you're putting in a higher quality fuel for your body that has some nutritional value, not just empty calories that you get from the Snickers bar. These two different foods are not going to have the same effect on your body when digested. Common sense will tell you that. How anyone could have thought of the term a calorie is a calorie is a calorie is beyond comprehension.

When it comes to calories, if you are counting those little bad boys, then my personal recommendation is to never go below 1500 calories a day, unless your doctor says otherwise. To me, anything below that is just too strict. If you are going to go super strict on calories, I also suggest taking vitamin and mineral supplements so your body can still operate efficiently, and your health doesn't take too big of a hit while consuming smaller portions of food. Also, I want to point out that the more physical you are or the more you work out, the more calories you can eat and still successfully lose weight.

If you are trying to shed some pounds and count calories in the process, keep this in mind; one pound of fat equals approximately 3500 calories.[46] Knowing that, if you do some simple math, then you'll realize that having a calorie deficit, whether it be by dieting, working out, or a combination of the two of 500 calories a day means you will lose one pound a week. A deficit of 1000 a day will lose you two pounds a week. Losing one to two pounds a week is the ideal rate.[47] That may sound slow, but it will add up over time pretty quickly. Slow and steady is the best way to shred fat and keep it off; when you lose too fast, it's usually a result of overtraining, or severely undereating, neither of which is sustainable. Remember the tortoise and the hare, slow and steady always wins the race. A bit cliché, but the world of fat loss still works on these same core principles, even if science teaches us new things we didn't know before. I'll leave you with this final piece of advice about diet.

I never recommend to anyone a kind of diet that you cannot do for the rest of your life. My advice is to not stress so much about things like counting calories and being precise on everything with your diet. Although, if you want to count calories and measure out all your food, then that's great! You can certainly do that and it will only benefit you. However, what I stress more about than the fine details is having good diet habits like the ones I've mentioned. Don't eat too close to bed, have good portion control, eat slowly, five small meals a day, a protein with every meal, load up on veggies, only allow once in a while cheat meals, and stay hydrated. Embracing these habits and making it part of a healthy lifestyle will take you very far. Even though I'm not a big advocate for counting calories, it's not a bad idea to keep a food journal, at least at first until you can develop good strong diet habits. Maintaining a food journal will help you see what and how much you are truly eating throughout the day.[48] The benefit of this is that this can help you spot some potential bad habits so you can recognize them and implement some changes to correct them, and a food journal also helps you stay accountable, which is huge.[48] Now the problem when it comes to being overly strict with your diet is that I find with this kind of dieting, or fad diets are that they are only temporary diets, and can hurt you in the long run without incredible discipline.

What I see too often is someone goes on a very restrictive diet that is astoundingly difficult to maintain for a very long time, then they end up going off the diet and binging. Being too restrictive with your diet can cause your body to go into starvation mode and start eating away at muscle tissue, rather than the intended fat.[49] Since your body is losing muscle your base metabolic rate decreases, and as soon as you go back to a normal diet your metabolism is slower than it was before, and unable to burn as many calories at the same rate you were able to before you naturally gain all the weight back you may have lost, and potentially put on even more, especially if you end up binging.[49] This can be incredibly frustrating, but entirely avoidable. I believe if you start incorporating my advice you won't have to worry about going on any fad diets, or crazy restrictive diets that will leave you hungry, tired, and in the long-term, not likely any farther ahead; and maybe even be in worse shape than when you started.

Chapter Nine Summary:

- **When it comes to how you look, diet trumps your workouts. Eighty percent of your appearance is related to diet, twenty percent is physical activity.**

- **A common misconception: if you work out you can eat whatever you want. This is false. An hour of hard work in the gym can be destroyed by the five minutes it takes to eat that piece of cheesecake.**

- Diet becomes more prevalent to your appearance as you age, in part due to the slowing of your metabolism.

- Food is fuel for your workouts. The better the fuel, the better the workouts, which equates to better results.

- Food can be your medicine or your poison.

- Not just what you eat matters, volume matters too. Even too much healthy food can make you fat.

- Five small meals a day is better than three big ones. Eating every few hours keeps your blood sugar and energy levels more stable, all of which is better for the waistline.

- Eat a protein with every meal. Protein digests slower than carbs. Fat and fiber digest the slowest. Complex carbs from fruits and veggies digest slower than simple carbs, such as sugar.

- For those looking to gain muscle, eat one gram of protein per pound of body weight.

- Avoid fruit juice if you're looking to lose weight. Instead of apple juice, eat an apple. Instead of orange juice, eat an orange, etc. You get much slower digesting fiber with whole fruit than just the sugary juice.

- Sugar is much worse to consume than fat, both for health and body weight reasons. Healthy fats are in things like fish or nuts.

- It's better to eat whole foods in general and not processed garbage. Vegetables are better for you eaten raw. You get more nutrients that way. If you cook them, steamed veggies are the best way to cook them.

- Don't eat less than three hours before bedtime. Food will mostly be stored as fat while you sleep. Don't work out too close to bedtime either. This will stimulate you and could disturb your sleep.

- Eat slowly; it can take twenty minutes before your brain signals you are full.

- Limit simple carbs such as bread or junk food. Focus on complex carbs from fruits and veggies. Veggies should be consumed more than other foods. About fifty percent of daily food intake should come from plant-based foods.

- Cheat meals aren't needed for your body but can give you a mental break from the high pressure of eating clean for long periods of time.

- Eating right at least eighty percent of the time should result in body changes.

- It's better to weed out bad foods and only indulge once in a while than to cut them out cold turkey to lessen severe cravings.

Your taste buds can be retrained over time.

- If you crave sweets, reach for some fruit.

- Your workout can affect your appetite. Weights can increase appetite, cardio suppresses.

- Fluid intake is of extreme importance. Always stay hydrated. Ignore the drink eight; eight-ounce glasses a day rule. Your hydration needs depend on three things: your weight, activity level, and climate. Half to one ounce of water per pound of body weight is a good rule of thumb.

- Hydration levels can affect performance in the gym. If you're dehydrated your workouts will suffer.

- The term a calorie is a calorie is a calorie is crap! Yes, fewer calories in than out will result in weight loss in a normal healthy body, but the better quality calories, the better healthy body.

- Below fifteen hundred calories a day is too extreme. Stay above this if you're trying to lose weight. The more active you are the more calories you can consume.

- One pound of fat equals approximately thirty-five hundred calories.

- Losing one to two pounds of body fat a week is ideal. Losing weight too fast rarely results in long-term success.

- Never start a diet regimen you can't do the rest of your life. Fad diets are just that, their fads.

- Good diet habits: don't eat too close to bed, have good portion control, eat slowly, five small meals a day, a protein with every meal, load up on veggies, only allow once in a while cheat meals, and stay hydrated.

- **A food journal can be a useful tool.**

Chapter Ten: *Put the Couch Away!*

Lesson 10: Take short breaks in between exercises.

The time you spend in the gym is precious, so don't waste it. I've seen it time and time again, and have done it myself occasionally as well; people will take far too long of rest breaks in between their sets or exercises. This all relates to your intensity and limiting distractions in the first chapter as well. Taking too long of breaks will prevent you from seeing eye-popping results. It can dial your intensity down to a level too low to cause any serious change to your body. Remember, it must be hard in order for it to take you to the next level of fitness and get anything noticeable out of your workouts. If it doesn't challenge you how can it change you? To a certain point of extremism, the harder it is, the better it is. Resting too much will slow your heart rate and will cause much less muscle fiber to engage in the movements you're doing.[50] The lower your break times are, the more muscle fibers that will end up being engaged, which is going to give you the kind of results you want.[50] What happens when you rest your muscles too much is that your body doesn't need to recruit other muscle fibers that are not fatigued, and so you are not developing nearly as much muscle as you could.[50] Also, if you rest too much you risk cooling your body down, and in doing so you risk injury. Plus, the fact that your heart rate drops most likely means you're burning fewer calories. It's just bad all around.

I see this mistake quite a lot, and I've been guilty of this blunder as well. I think part of the problem for some people is once it starts getting hard they let off the gas because of the discomfort it's causing them. There have been times when this was definitely the case for me. Rather than pushing through the intense discomfort, I took a load off because I just didn't like what I was experiencing. On the other hand, I've had serious determination and grit at times to the point of even being called crazy, a good crazy, though. You have to fight the temptation to ease up. Pushing through barriers on a progressive level is going to get you to where you want to go. And in order to get better at something you have to at the very least attempt to push yourself to a point you haven't reached yet. You have to do what you have not done before. If you want to get better at pull-ups and be able to do more than you could the last time you did pullups, you have to push yourself to try that one more pull-up. The strength and endurance changes will come it just takes time and effort.

Generally speaking, unless you are doing some seriously intense weight lifting, you should try to keep your breaks to under a minute.[50] Shorter breaks will keep your heart rate elevated; you'll burn more calories, and this will give you a much more intense quality workout. Only if you are doing some serious power lifting should you take more than one minute, but not more than three minutes.[52] The reason being is that the muscle fibers that are used in power moves will naturally take longer to recuperate.[51] However, after a few minutes, your muscles start to get cold again, and you're not pushing them hard enough to cause growth or change. You're also increasing your chance of injury.

Try to time your breaks by using a stopwatch or by watching the clock on the gym wall. It may seem tedious, but if you break it down to a science, it's only going to make your workouts that much more effective. Now with that being said, I want to point out that there are three main types of muscle fibers in the human body, and they each serve a different purpose and require different amounts of rest. The three types are Type I, Type IIA, and Type IIB.[52]

Type I muscle fibers are referred to as your slow twitch fibers, Type IIA is your fast twitch fibers, and Type IIB falls in between Type I and Type IIA.[52] Your slow twitch muscle fibers engage in lower intensity movements, such as simple tasks.[52] These fibers have a lot of endurance and recuperate quicker than your fast twitch.[51] Therefore exercises that require more moderate intensity, or when you're working small muscle groups, you need less rest. The fast twitch fibers are your bigger muscle fibers, which use more force and require more rest to fully recuperate.[51] Hence the reason why if you are doing high intensity lifting it's a not a bad thing to rest up more in between sets. Otherwise, you will fatigue too quickly and won't be able to work your muscles to the full extent possible. The main thing to watch out for is to simply not take too long of breaks. This mistake is a very typical because it is easy to simply take an extended breather. If you want the work to count for something avoid this error, and it will undoubtedly make a difference in your results.

Chapter Ten Summary:

- **Longer rest breaks mean lower intensity levels.**

- **If it doesn't challenge you, how can it change you?**

- **Shorter break times means more muscle fibers engaged.**

- **Too long of breaks can cool the body down, which increases the risk of injury, and lowers the calories being burnt.**

- In order to get better at something, you have to at least attempt to push yourself to a point you haven't reached yet.

- Generally, try to keep your break times between sets/exercises under a minute.

- There are three main muscle fiber types: Type I, Type IIA, and Type IIB. Type I are slow twitch fibers, which engage in lower intense movements, have lots of endurance and recuperate quicker than fast twitch fibers. Type IIA are fast twitch fibers. These are bigger muscle fibers, which use more force and require more rest to fully recuperate. Type IIB fibers fall in between Type I and Type IIA.

Chapter Eleven: *Hey Buddy!*

Lesson 11: Utilize a support system/and or a workout buddy.

Going solo in the gym can be an extremely challenging undertaking. Unless you are extremely self-motivated, not having a workout partner or some kind of support system from friends and family; you will have a very tough time staying motivated for the long haul. You may join the gym with the very best intentions and feel extremely motivated in the beginning. What can and does often happen though is either you experience burnout or life gets in the way, and you shift your focus elsewhere. I can completely relate to life happening, and feeling as though time just isn't on your side to take the trip to the gym. Now, I would never advocate skipping a funeral, or something extremely important just to go to the gym. That would be foolish and wrong. However, having the support and push you need, or ideally a workout buddy for the times you can make it to the gym or do a workout, is vital. You need that support for the times you just don't feel like going to the gym. If you don't have the support you need, your chances of staying with your exercise program for the long-term are minuscule. I don't say that to be discouraging; I say it because it's true.

People need the support of others; it's a fact we cannot deny no matter how independent and strong we think we are. Going solo in any venture very seldom ends in success. Think of it this way; almost any successful person will tell you they had a mentor, a team behind them, or some help along the way to their success. These same people will likely tell you that they would not have made it on their own, or without some guidance or support system. That's another truth. Utilizing support mostly for psychological reasons, in my opinion, is essential. Having support will be a tremendous asset in helping you push past your barriers. The times that I've had the most success in the gym is when I've had a workout buddy, or been a part of a support group.

As of right now, I'm currently in a fitness support group, and I'm doing extremely well meeting my weekly goals. I honestly don't think I'd be having nearly as much success without the support I have and the motivation that the support group provides through our friendly competition. I'm a highly competitive individual, and that is one of the best ways to motivate me. I love it. I thrive on trying to be the best. I wouldn't consider myself a prideful person, but I like to win. I'm in no way a sore loser. If someone beats me, I tip my cap and move on, but victory drives me. I think this is in part why I'm a good athlete. I love the competition. They may say winning isn't everything, but without a drive to win, what is the point? If nobody wanted to win sports or any other kind of competitive event, they would be a bore to watch. It's just not fun without a challenge. I'm not saying you can't wing it and go to the gym on your own self-motivation. Some people do that and still do very well, but highly self-motivated individuals are a rare breed. Even the most self-motivated people will have their days where they just do not want to hit the gym. It's in these times where having support from others comes in and tackles that momentary weakness.

Thinking that you will never need support is a gym blunder that you must avoid. I've made this mistake before, and to be one-hundred percent honest, I've fallen short every time I've tried to do the gym thing entirely solo. I've had the least amount of success in the gym during these times, and the most success on the flip side of that coin; having a partner or a support system in place to back me up on the days I'm seriously struggling with my motivation. It's impossible for a human being to be on one-hundred percent of the time. You will have your off days. One day you might feel like a million bucks, the next day it feels like the weight of the world is bearing down on you and the gym is the last thing on your mind. Nobody is a machine, and nobody is perfect. Reach for perfection, but seek the support you need. As much as some of us may hate to admit, we all need to lean on each other from time to time.

Chapter Eleven Summary:

- Not having support from friends, family, or a workout partner makes long-term gym success extremely difficult.

- People need the support of others. This is a fact of human nature.

- Almost any successful person in any field had a mentor or some kind of support system that helped them along the way.

Chapter Twelve: *Wait a minute! Or Five*

Lesson 12: Skipping a warm up can lead to injury, and lower performance.

If you've ever experienced a serious injury that kept you from working out for any length of time, then you know how frustrating that can be. Knowing that, you'd never want to skip a warm up because that's one of the best ways that you can put yourself at the highest risk of injury. Not warming up before a workout is similar to taking a piece of gum and trying to stretch it before you've chewed on it and getting it wet.[53] If you try to stretch a dry piece of gum, we all know it'll rip apart. On the other hand, if you've chewed on a piece of gum you can stretch that sucker pretty far. Think of a piece of gum representing your muscle fibers. You can literally rip your muscle fibers right apart if you don't properly warm up and go right into a hard workout doing an intense movement right away.[53] It's not worth the five minutes you'll save by skipping a warm up. Those five minutes you've saved may put you on the couch for weeks, or even months if you tear something badly enough.

Warming up and cooling down has its purpose. When it comes to cooling down, a mere few minutes for some stretches and light movements will contribute greatly towards the beginning of your recovery between workouts, and bringing your heart rate down at a reasonable pace.[54] You don't want to just suddenly stop working out after getting your heart rate up there, that can cause complications, possibly even makes you suddenly pass out. The science behind that is this: when you work out your blood vessels expand. If you suddenly stop moving (which helps keep the blood flowing) then what can happen is blood will pool in your leg muscles and not be able to be pumped up to the rest of your body, hence causing you to pass out.[54] And that you most definitely do not want to happen. Now when it comes to warming up, there is a dual purpose to it. Injury prevention is the most important reason to warm up.[55] The other reason is for the simple fact warming up is preparing your body to do work.[55]

Warming up can boost your performance just for the simple fact you properly got your body ready before you did your first official exercise of the workout. [56]

One thing I have to mention about warming up. The old school way of thinking was that warming up should include some static stretching of the muscles you're going to use. For example, if you are going to work your chest muscles, do chest stretches, and static stretching meaning you're only holding the stretch, there's no movement involved while you do the stretch. Recent research has shown that doing this kind of stretching can actually decrease your performance.[57] Instead, you should do ballistic stretching during warm up, and only do static stretches either after the workout or during the workout in between exercises after you are fully warmed up and engaged in your workout.[57] Ballistic stretching is stretching that involves moving through the stretch, not just holding the stretch.[58] A good example would be if you are trying to stretch your chest muscles you could swing your arms back and forth from front to back. When you're swinging your arms towards your back, you would feel the stretch. It's stretching the muscles but at the same time, it's a light warm up because it involves movement. This kind of stretching is fine to do as part of a warmup.

A proper warm-up can be done in one of two ways. First, you can do some light cardio such as a light jog on the treadmill for about five to ten minutes.[56] Getting your heart rate up and the blood flowing through your body is going to warm your muscles up, so they are ready for the pounding you're about to give them. Another way you can warm up your muscles is to do some light exercises using the same muscles you will be using during the actual workout.[56] For example, if you're going to be working out your arms with some weight training, then you could warm them up by doing some bicep curls with a light weight. The light bicep curls will get your muscles ready for that kind of movement, and of course, they will get the blood flowing to those specific muscles to get them warm. You can warm up either one of these ways, and that's perfectly fine, or you can do a combination of both.

As long as you do a warm up for at least a few minutes, you should be okay. I recommend a minimum of five minutes; that should be a good enough warm up to help decrease the chances of injury and to reap the benefits of better performing muscles during your workout. You don't need to go crazy with the warm up and spend twenty minutes running on the treadmill. I see some people do some exercises that they consider a warm up, when in reality; it's an actual workout, not a warm up. Not warming up is another easily preventable gym blunder. Ease into the workout with your warmups; they will help you get the job done safely, and more efficiently.

Chapter Twelve Summary:

- **Skipping a warm up is one of the best ways to increase the chance of injury.**

- **The cooldown has its place too. A mere few minutes of stretches and light movements** starts the recovery process and lowers the heart rate at a reasonable pace.

- Warm up isn't just for injury prevention. It prepares your body to do work and can boost performance.

- Static stretching during warm up has been shown to decrease performance. Ballistic stretching is more effective.

- A proper warm up can be simply doing some light cardio or doing light exercises that use the same muscles to be used during the workout.

- A minimum of five minutes is recommended for the warm up.

Chapter Thirteen: *Write It Down!*

Lesson 13: Plan and track your workouts.

Failing to plan means planning for failure. Most of us have probably heard that little piece of advice, and it's positively correct. It's true with most things in life. It's certainly true in business. Most business owners that just wing it without a solid business plan fail. That's one of the biggest reasons why businesses fail; because they don't have a plan to achieve the goals that they need to reach to thrive. Most of us have planned to fail by not planning in our personal lives, too. You've got to have a plan, and when it comes to your workouts, it's no different. Just winging it is not the way to go. You don't have to break it down to an exact science, and most don't, but if you're going to the gym without a real idea of your goals and how it is you are going to achieve these aims, chances are you won't be seeing much changes with your body. Plan your workouts ahead of time. Write everything down and track your progress, and results. How do you know where it is you want to go if you don't know where you have been?

Writing down and tracking everything you do with your workouts will help you see progress over time, and it will certainly assist you in your goal setting. I love seeing gains, both in the mirror and on paper where I am able to see how much I've progressed over time. I'm a stats guy. Stats fascinate me, which is probably one of the reasons why I'm such a huge baseball fan, which is the most stat-driven sport ever invented. Seeing my own stats reveal how I've improved, for example, on my bench press, gives me great satisfaction and a sense of pride. It also lets me set a mark, or goal. For example, one goal could be something along the lines of; to be able to lift a certain amount of weight doing bicep curls by a certain amount of time, and then reward myself when achieving that goal. It is my opinion that those who don't write their workout plans and results down, or at the very least track their workouts in some fashion, don't reach the best results that they have the potential to reach. The standard advice on how to achieve your personal goals, no matter what it is, is first to write it down.[59] It's been proven time and time again that those who do write their goals down, and what exactly it is they need to do to reach those goals, are the most successful people at attaining them. And remember to reward yourself for achieving your goals.

Other than the satisfaction of chiseling an amazing body, which takes time, you want to have some satisfaction in reaching each and every one of your mini-goals leading up to the end results. My advice is to make your rewards something tangible that will last. Buy something you've wanted to for a while. It's ok to splurge on yourself once in a while, especially when it is a reward for hitting a goal in the gym, which makes it more meaningful. However, I never recommend rewarding yourself with food. For one thing, food is very temporary. The satisfaction from food only lasts for a few minutes, often followed by guilt if you reward yourself with junk. At least that's been my experience when rewarding myself in that fashion. Reward yourself with something that will give you lasting satisfaction, such as a new pair of shoes, an outfit, a movie you've wanted to buy, or whatever it is that you desire. You could even reward yourself with an experience. What I mean by that is say there's a rock band you want to see, go buy some tickets. That's just one example. Be creative in rewarding yourself, food is too simple in my opinion. Even though I have an intense love for food, something that is certainly a cause for my struggles with diet, I just don't feel that food is a great reward, for anything really. And finally, don't' make the mistake of shooting in the dark with no plan of action. Heed this advice and your chances of success will soar.

Chapter Thirteen Summary:

- **Not planning means planning for failure.**

- **If you're going to the gym without a real idea of your goals and how it is you are going to achieve them, chances are you won't be seeing much for results.**

- Write everything down. Track your progress and results. Seeing your results in the mirror and on paper can be very motivating.

- It's been proven time and time again that those who write their goals down, and what it is exactly they need to do to achieve them are the most successful people at attaining them.

- Reward yourself when you reach a goal. Make the reward something tangible and long lasting, not something temporary like food.

Chapter Fourteen: *The Order of Things*

Lesson 14: Weights first, then cardio. Bigger muscles first, then smaller.

You may not think the order in which you do your exercises in your workout matter, but there's some science that says that it does. A lot of people do both weight/strength training, and cardio; which is great because in doing so you're working both your skeletal muscular system and your heart and lungs. Working all systems of the body will lead you to the best fitness levels. However, for those who choose to do both a weight training session and a cardio session on the same day, and many times in succession, some make the mistake of doing cardio first, then weight training. This is the opposite of how you want to be structuring your workouts. There's more than one reason for the thinking behind this.

Starting your workout session with cardio before weights may fatigue you to the point that your weight training will not be as effective as it could be.[60] Some may argue that if you do weight training first, then you'll be too fatigued for a good cardio session. That's not normally the case, and in fact, doing weights first can help warm your body up for cardio.[60] Even though weight training can certainly make you feel fatigued; weight training is an anaerobic exercise, one that does not require oxygen, but instead uses internal energy sources, such as glycogen (stored carbohydrates),[62] blood sugar, or fat.[61] These energy sources can become strained in shorter periods of time than when you are performing a cardio session. The reason being is that cardio is an aerobic exercise, meaning it requires oxygen, and of course, oxygen is plentiful unless you are working out at a high altitude.[61]

Although doing cardio can dip into other energy sources such as fat, it's not as intense on your skeletal muscles, but it is more intense for your heart and lungs. This is one reason why it is better to do weights first then cardio if you're doing both kinds of training on the same day, especially if you are doing weights then cardio right after. If you are doing them in succession, I do recommend giving yourself a few minutes break after your weight training before you start your cardio training. The reason being is when you do weight training you will get a "pump," which means blood has engorged the muscles you've worked, which makes them look "pumped up," hence where the term comes from.[63] You should give your body a few minutes for some of the blood to leave the pumped-up muscles so your body can distribute the blood to other parts of the body where it will be needed more when you are doing your cardio. Of course, if you take a decent size break in between your weight session and cardio you will want to do another light warm up and then begin your cardio, so as to lower your chances of injury.

The other reason for doing weights first is for the simple fact that it typically takes your body about twenty minutes of exercising before it begins to tap into your fat stores.[64] Since cardio is a better form of exercise to burning fat than weights, it naturally makes sense to do cardio after because you will have started to use your stored fat energy sources by the time your cardio session begins. This will cause you to burn the most fat, and in my opinion, that's always a good thing. Now when it comes to what kind of exercises you should do first, this also does matter; more so when it comes to weight training does the order of which types of exercises you do matter.

Typically, it is better to first do the most complicated moves or ones that require multiple muscle groups, bigger muscle groups and muscle fibers to engage.[65] If you are working both big and small muscle groups on the same day, it makes much more sense to work the larger muscle groups first; for example, back and biceps.[65] Back muscles would be considered the big muscle group, while biceps are the smaller muscle group. Back and biceps are a good example because a lot of back exercises require you to use your biceps as a supporting muscle group in most back exercises. For example, while doing a pull-up, the primary muscles you're working are your lats, but your biceps assist in the movement as well, it's just not the muscle group that is getting the most focus out of the exercise. If you were to do all your biceps exercises first and "pre-fatigue" your biceps and then work your back; you are not going to be able to perform as well while working your back because your assisted muscles, the biceps, are already fatigued. For these reasons you will not be able to do the most effective workout you can, and as I've pointed out before, that means fewer results. I've seen this kind of mistake many times.

This principle is the same with all muscle groups. Keep in mind the big muscle groups are your back, chest, and legs (quads, hamstrings, and glutes). The small muscle groups are your shoulders, arms, your core (abs, side oblique's, and lower back), and your calve muscles.[66] So keep this in mind when you are working different muscles in your workouts.

Chapter Fourteen Summary:

- **The order of your exercises matter. Weight training should be done before cardio.**

- **Cardio first can cause fatigue to the point that weight training performance will suffer. Weights will warm your body up and you'll be better prepared for cardio. Cardio isn't as intense on your skeletal muscles like weights are; it's more intense for your heart and lungs.**

- **If you're doing weights and cardio on the same day give yourself at least a few minutes of rest before starting cardio after weights.**

- **It typically takes about twenty minutes for your body to dip into fat reserves when exercising. Cardio is better for fat burning so weights first, in this case, makes sense for better fat loss.**

- It's better to work big muscles first than small. Often the small muscles assist the bigger muscles in the more complex movements. Pre-fatiguing the small assisting muscles first will cause a lack of performance on the more complex movements that require the bigger muscle to engage with assistant from the smaller muscles. Doing bicep curls before pullups (which works your back with assistance from the smaller bicep muscles) is a good example. This will result in a less effective workout.

- Big muscle groups: Back, chest, and legs (quads, hamstrings, and glutes.)

- Small muscle groups: Shoulders, arms, (biceps, triceps), your core (abs, side oblique's, and lower back), and calves.

Chapter Fifteen: *Tid Bits of Fit*

Lesson 15: A collection of helpful tips and useful knowledge.

Up to this point, this book has primarily been about the common mistakes that I see people making in the gym, but I also want you to get a good grasp on the things that you should be doing as well. This chapter is entirely devoted to showing you some helpful tips and useful knowledge that will aid you in the quest for your perfect body. Couple this information with knowing the kinds of mistakes you should be avoiding; and you will be armed to the gills with a ton of knowledge and insight that will help you get the results that we all crave when making appearance after appearance at the gym. This collection of tid bits of fit are what I believe are the most pertinent tips and knowledge you can use.

Remember the acronym "FITT":

If you are doing well with your diet, have no underlying medical conditions that can make changing your body composition difficult, or impossible, and you are still not getting results, the easiest way to figure out a possible explanation as to why is to remember the four main criteria affecting the quality of your workouts. The acronym FITT stands for Frequency, Intensity, Time, and Type of exercise.[67] You have to make a change to either one of these criteria, or a combination of some, or all of these if your results are not coming through.[67] Here, the four main criteria are broken down.

Frequency: This is simply the number of times you are working out in a given period of time, such as a week.[67] As I previously mentioned, I don't' recommend working out seven days a week because your body's need for rest is crucial, but at the same time if you're only working out just one or two days a week; that's not going to result in much if any change. You should be working out at a bare minimum of three to four times a week, but no more than six days a week.[67]

Intensity: In my opinion, this is the most important aspect of any quality workout. Intensity is the most common element that needs to be changed for people to reach their fitness goals. Laziness is a nasty goal busting habit. Be not lazy; let your hard work shine through.

Time: You can't expect to get anywhere if you only spend a few minutes working out each time you go to the gym. Generally speaking the more intense the workout, the shorter it can be, but a good rule of thumb is thirty to sixty minutes in the gym is plenty. And the total accumulated time you spend working out each day doesn't necessarily have to be in one sitting. You can split your workouts into different time slots each day, but make sure each workout is at least ten minutes long. Anything less won't reap you much for benefits.[68]

Type of exercise: Periodically mix up your workouts and exercises you are doing or you'll plateau. Plateauing sucks the motivation right out of you. It feels like hard work with no reward. Over time no one can withstand that kind of defeat. A good rule of thumb, mix up your routine at least every six weeks or less.

Intensity Techniques:

Here is a list of tips and techniques on how you can up your intensity game. Since lack of intensity is what I believe to be the number one reason why some people do not see results from the work they put in the gym, here are some ways you can improve the intensity of your workouts that will make them worthwhile, and cause a noticeable change.

Cardio/strength training intensity:

High-intensity interval training, aka "HIIT," is something most of us have probably heard of by now. In a nutshell, HIIT training is working out in intervals of high intensity followed by short periods rest.[69] A good example of this is a Tabata - style workout. An example of that would be sprinting as hard as you can for twenty seconds, followed by ten seconds of rest/light movement, and doing this for several cycles.[71] This style of workout I believe is much, much more effective than steady state cardio. A good example of steady state cardio is spending thirty minutes jogging on a treadmill, or using an elliptical at the same speed and difficulty for the entire duration of the workout.[70] It's just one continuous movement that doesn't go up or down in intensity. This style of workout can get incredibly boring, and is far less effective than dialing the intensity up with a HIIT style workout.[71] HIIT workouts are an excellent way to increase the intensity of your workouts, especially when it comes to cardio.

Bodybuilding/weight training intensity:

If you are more interested in say
bodybuilding style workouts, or just weight training
in general, than you have several techniques at your
disposal that can increase the intensity of those style
of workouts. Here is a list with a description of each.

Manipulate Time/Add weight:

The most basic way you can increase the
intensity of your workouts is to take shorter breaks
in between sets/exercises, and or add weight.[72]
Taking shorter breaks in between exercises or sets
will increase your endurance over time. Endurance
is a huge area of fitness that you want to improve if
you want to get the best results. The better your
endurance is, the higher quality workouts you can
muster through. Adding weight will naturally
increase the intensity of your workout by making it
harder.[72] Increase weight slowly, but progressively.
However, know your limits. Increase the amount of
weight you do at a level that you know your body

can safely handle. Only you can truly determine that. Your body will adapt over time and what felt heavy at first will feel light over time (within limits), but the human body is only capable of lifting so much weight, so don't go too crazy with increasing weight.

Muscle Confusion:

This technique is pretty straightforward. Your muscles need to be confused from time to time. Doing the same routine over and over again will result in the dreaded plateau. Since our bodies are amazing at adaptation, muscle confusion is a necessary element of gym success. You can do this in a variety of ways. Mix up or change your routine from time to time, lift heavier weights/increase the intensity of cardio moves, take shorter breaks, do more reps than usual, do your routine in an unfamiliar order, increase the speed/tempo of your workout, doing new exercises you haven't done before, or do any of the other intensity techniques mentioned in this chapter.

Rest/Pause (Forced) Reps:

Most of the time what you see in the gym is someone lifting a weight a certain number of reps, or a maximum number of reps until they can't do even one more rep (the proper method). But it is possible for you to go even further than that with this technique. Once you've done your last rep and you can't perform even one more rep, take a quick three to five-second breather and do another rep, or two, or as many as you can until your body doesn't allow you to do another.[72] You can continue to do this a few times, and this will exponentially increase the intensity of your workout.

Partial Reps:

Partial reps are a good technique you can combine with forced reps if choose to. When you have fatigued yourself to the point that you can't complete even one more rep in a full range of motion; than do some reps as far as you physically can.[72] A good example of this would be if you're doing bicep curls and you're at the point you can't lift the dumbbells all the way to your shoulder; then lift it as far as you can until you literally can't lift it at all. Example: if you can only lift the dumbbells half way up to your shoulder then do so. You will get to the point where you can't raise the weights at all, and then you can take a normal break, or bang out some forced reps in the same fashion as I pointed out in the previous intensity technique. Don't worry if people will come up to you and tell you that you're doing it wrong and that you are supposed to lift the weight in the full range of motion. Yes, full range of motion is of utmost importance. However, when you've done all you can in the full range of motion, and you can only do partial reps, you will get way more intensity out of your workouts. As a bonus, you will very likely get better results than the advice givers will simply for their lack of knowledge.

Isolation Training:

Isolation training means to train each individual muscle group separately.[72] Isolation training is a simple concept. It's the opposite of doing compound movements, which work multiple muscle groups at the same time,[72] which yes I recommend doing, but training each muscle group separately in addition to performing compound movements will help give you a more defined look.[72] A good example of a compound movement vs. an isolation movement would be doing pushups, or bench presses vs. dumbbell flys. Push ups and bench presses may primarily be a chest exercise, but you have to use other supporting muscle groups in the process of doing these types of exercises. You incidentally work your shoulders and triceps as well as your pecs when doing bench press. Same thing with pushups, with the addition of working your core muscles to keep your body up off the ground. A pec isolation move would be the dumbbell flys. Doing that particular move makes you focus much more directly on the chest without much effort needed from your supporting muscle groups.

Negative Reps:

As I've pointed out earlier in this book, the negative motion of an exercise does more for you than the positive. The negative motion of a bicep curl is when you are letting the weight down, positive when you curl it up. A neat way to increase your intensity is through the use of the negative portion of the rep, and to do it very slowly. There are a few different scenarios where you can utilize.

On the negative rep of a bicep curl, you simply let it down very slowly. Trust me when I say you will feel it, and you will fatigue very quickly, which is a good thing. Another way you can do this is to take a very heavy weight, more than you can currently do (enlist the help of a spotter if need be) and then lower the weight as slow as you can for as many reps as you can. This unique technique will boost your strength and give you amazing results. I like doing this with bench presses. It's a great way to increase strength and add intensity. Finally, another method is to have your partner slowly press down on the weight as you resist against his pushing while lowering the weights as slowly as you can. The combination of the weight itself and your partner pushing down on the weight will up your intensity to the max. This kind of negative rep is also known as forced negatives.[72]

The Cheating Method:

The cheating method is one of my personal favorite intensity techniques. Cheating (with a purpose) can cause some heads to turn your way, but trust me, ignore them; they simply don't know what you are doing. With this method be especially careful not to do overdo it this is an advanced move. The cheating method goes like this. I'll use the bicep curl again as the example. Say you do eight reps with absolute strict form, and you simply can't do rep number nine with strict proper form. With this method, the idea is to cheat (incorporate other muscles) just enough so you can do a few more reps.[72] The idea isn't to make it easier, but to force the target muscles (biceps) to do more work even though they've been thoroughly exhausted.[72] By cheating, or swinging the weight up just barely enough so you can do a rep you are still forcing your bicep to do work beyond the kind of stress you would normally put on your muscles by doing just strict form styled reps, even while incorporating other muscles like your back or shoulder muscles. The cheating method is an excellent technique for breaking through plateaus.

Drop Sets:

I love doing drop sets. This technique is another favorite of mine. Drop sets are simple and very effective in my opinion. I'll go to my favorite example again too, the bicep curl. A drop set would entail the following; while doing bicep curls, you do as many reps as you can to failure. After you can't do any more reps then lower (drop) the amount of weight and then do more reps at the lighter weight until failure.[72] You can add several drop sets to one exercise. An example of this would be what's called running the rack. What I mean by this is starting off with a heavier weight that's sitting on a weight rack, and then doing as many drop sets as it takes to get to the lightest weight.[72] Drop sets are an excellent intensity increasing technique! Your muscles will be extremely pumped and fatigued, all of which is a good thing.

Supersets/Giant Sets/Circuits:

A superset would be when you do one exercise and then do another different exercise immediately afterward with no rest in between.[72] You can do this for the same muscle group, or do an exercise for one muscle group and then a different one. An example of this for the same muscle group would be doing a set of bench presses for your chest, and then with no rest in between doing dumbbell flys, which also works the chest, but at a different angle. An example of combining different muscle groups with a superset would be doing bench presses for a set, then working your back with something like pull-ups immediately after with no rest. A giant set is the same idea, but with three back to back to back exercises rather than just two. A circuit would be doing this principle with four or more exercises back to back with no rest.

Ballistic Training:

Ballistic training is an interesting way to increase intensity in your workout. Ballistic training is what I would refer to as using explosiveness, or power to finish an exercise movement. I will use the leg press exercise as an example. The way to do a ballistic move or training while doing a leg press would be to lower the weight (the negative movement) at a reasonable speed, then explode the weight up (positive movement) as hard and fast as you can, but controlled and safely.[72] Ballistic training is different than regular training where you are doing your exercises at one constant speed. This technique is fantastic for training for power, and you can implement it in almost any kind of exercise.

Sleep and Rest Days:

If only us humans could evolve to the point where we don't need the standard eight hours of sleep to function at full capacity, or need sleep at all. Imagine how much we could accomplish, but alas you can't fight against human nature, and win. Besides, in my opinion, sleep is rather great. When I can sleep, and sleep well, it's lovely. And when it comes to the gym, sleep is much more important than most give it credit for. Sleeping is necessary for healing and change to take place in your body.[73] It's ridiculously important. The time that you are sleeping is the time when your body does the most muscle repair and building, and therefore the time when your body adapts and becomes stronger than it was before to help you meet the demands you previously placed on your body.[73] If you don't get enough rest, you will slow this process way down, and it can mess with your hormones too.

You will likely crave sweet stuff with too little sleep.[74] You can feel sluggish due to a slowing of your metabolism, which is bad in and of its own since you will burn fewer calories.[75] Also, we all know how it can put you in a foul mood, and let's face it, a foul mood isn't exactly when you will be feeling the most motivated and energetic, and ready to hit the gym. If you are on a bodybuilding regimen and trying to put on some mass, ZZZ's will get you inches. My simple advice, do your best to get your eight hours of sleep. If you are doing crazy intense exercises, it's not a bad idea to shoot for ten hours if you can. That can be very challenging in today's busy world, but you will feel all around better, and be able to perform better in the gym as well. Rest days off from the gym have their importance as well.

Even though you can technically do cardio every day if you wanted to, I recommend taking one day to give yourself a break and let your body recover as I previously mentioned. I also recommend that when you have finished through a cycle of a workout program, say one that was three months long, it's not a bad idea to take a small vacation from the gym. Even taking a week off periodically is not a bad idea. Taking a mini-vacation like this will help your body fully recover from the beating it's been taking. Most, if not all of us take vacations from our jobs, taking small breaks from working out, is good for you as well. It's good for your body and mind. Rest is high on the list of importance when it comes to the gym. Don't underestimate its importance.

The Dreaded Scale:

When it comes to weight loss and weighing yourself, I recommend only doing so once a week, or even less often than that. Try not to obsess over the number on the scale and end up weighing yourself every day, or more than once a week. Lasting change and weight loss is a slow process, and the results will be subtle, but if you do all the right things and follow the advice in this book, results will come, and you will see them in time on the scale, and more importantly, in the mirror. Obsessing over the scale is not going to make it happen faster, and it can be very frustrating and put undue stress on you when you only see tiny incremental changes, or worse, no changes at all, or your weight bounced back a little. That can be unsettling.

Keep in mind as well that it is perfectly normal for your weight to fluctuate within a few pounds up or down on a daily basis.[76] Fluctuation like this can be due to water retention, how much you've recently eaten, the lovely stuff in your bowels, and other factors;[76] so that means if you were to weigh yourself on a daily basis you could see a sudden jump in weight, and that could send you into a panic. We don't want that. The trick is to look for the trend; is your weight gradually going down, up, or hovering around the same few pounds? Let's say you weigh yourself once a week, and you have one week where you didn't lose anything, or even maybe gained a pound or two; this should not cause you to go into panic mode, look at the trend. If you were to draw a graph you might see some bumps in the road, but as long as the trend is downward, or in the direction you want it to be going then you know you are doing something right. No matter what the scale tells you, stay consistent with the efforts and the results will come along. Stay in the fight!

The best time to weigh yourself is in the am after you have gone the bathroom, and with little to no clothing.[76] Yes, even the smallest amount of clothing will add a surprising amount to your scale. Doing this is going to give you the closest real body weight because it's likely you will not be as bloated or full of bodily waste at that time. Given that, the worst time to weigh yourself is at night. In fact, during my time in the weight loss competition I recently had with some friends, we would always weigh ourselves Sunday night, but I would always weigh myself again Monday morning, and not again until the next Sunday evening. Almost every Sunday evening vs. Monday morning my weight was about two pounds less on Monday morning than Sunday evening. My thoughts on that; the cause was due to clothing weight (given the fact I didn't consider weighing myself naked in front of my friends), and bodily waste/fluid retention as well.

The scale is helpful in seeing if your weight loss efforts are paying off, or even weight/muscle gains, but the best tool to use in gauging your progress is the mirror. How you look as opposed to that dreaded scale is going to tell you much more about what's happening to your body. During weight loss, you could lose fat and gain muscle at the same time. Just looking at the scale is not going to tell you that, unless it has a built-in body fat analyzer. Just a regular handheld body fat analyzer can be a useful tool as well.

If you are trying to lose weight you certainly want to be losing fat, but not muscle. Holding onto muscle will keep your metabolism cranked up. As I've mentioned before, the amount of muscle you have will have a direct effect on your resting metabolism. It's going to hurt you, in the long run, to lose a bunch of weight quickly, just to regain it because you lost so much muscle in the process that your resting metabolism slowed way down. This is part of the reason why slow and steady weight loss will likely result in you keeping the weight off. People that starve themselves, or go crazy with the cardio while not eating enough will likely experience this problem. This is my belief as to why most of the contestants on weight loss TV shows end up regaining most if not all, and sometimes more weight than when they started the competition. They are losing weight way too fast, working out way too much, and causing too much muscle loss to occur right along with the fat. That is my opinion. If I'm right, what's happening is their metabolism ends up slowing to such a crawl that even eating a minuscule amount of food will make their bodies put that weight right back on.

Just losing fat and not muscle is ideal. If you are cutting your weight down its highly likely you will lose some muscle too, but try to keep it to a minimum by consuming plenty of protein.[77] Protein shakes are not a bad idea and do some resistant training as well to try and at least maintain the muscle you do have.[77] As I've mentioned before, one to two pounds lost a week should be your goal if you're trying to cut fat. Anything more and you risk losing too much muscle in the weight loss process. Remember the cliché; the tortoise always beats the hare, even in weight loss.

Lastly, I advise caution when you see all these ads that say you can lose an insane amount of weight in a short period of time. Stay away from them you don't need that in your life. If you truly want to lose the weight and keep it off, making slow incremental changes like losing two pounds a week is what will give you the lasting results you want.

The Beginnings of Weight loss:

It's useful to know that if you are embarking on a weight loss journey when you first start, your body is generally going to use up glycogen (stored carbohydrates in your muscles), and you will lose water weight before your body starts to tap into your fat reserves.[78] Because of this fact in the first week or two, maybe three, it's not uncommon for the amount of weight loss to be much higher than the recommended one to two pounds a week. However, after your body has gotten rid of the excess water, and used up stored glycogen your body will start to use its fat reserves, which will also mean the amount of weight you lose will be a smaller amount. This is not a bad thing; it just means you've gotten past the initial weight loss phase, and you're moving onto losing that fat you want to take off.

You can't Spot Reduce Fat:

There's a common misconception that if you want to reduce the fat on your tummy than just do a bunch of sit-ups or ab workouts. This is completely false. You can't just pick a body part and work that area of your body and end up losing fat in that same area.[78] It simply doesn't work that way. If only it did, we would see a lot more flat washboard abs out there. Not much if anything about achieving the body of your dreams is easy. Remember that. This is especially true if you want a six-pack to die for. Your body doesn't pull fat from where the work is being done to it. Generally, the body will pull fat in an order that is genetically instructed to do so for your body.[79] No two bodies are identical, so it really depends on your genetic makeup that you have no control over.[79] In most cases, your body will pull fat from all over your body, but because the most fat is usually stored in the gut area (especially for men);

this is why this area seems to lose fat last.[80] I also want to point out the different kinds of fat your body will burn over time.

In your body, there is visceral fat, subcutaneous fat, and internal fat in your muscles, joints, etc.[81,82] Visceral fat is internal fat that is stored in the gut area behind your ab muscles and is stored around your organs.[81] It's the unhealthiest fat that you can have in your body and is the reason for a protruding gut because it's behind the muscles pushing them outward.[81] Subcutaneous fat is fat that we see that's directly below the skin, and of course, you have your internal fat stored in muscles and different parts of the body.[81,82] You can't just choose where you want the fat to come off; you just have to keep dieting and working out until you get the desired results.

In some cases, it can take a bit of time before you will even begin to see any results whatsoever. It's not that uncommon to not see anything happening on the scale or mirror for the first six weeks of first starting a rigorous workout program designed to help you lose weight.[83] The reason for this is because when you are putting a sudden stress on the body with something like intense workouts, your muscles can react by holding onto water.[83] However, if you are still not seeing results after six weeks and you're doing everything correctly with diet and your workouts, it would be wise to consult with your doctor. I'm not a medical professional, but common resources will tell you that you could have an underlying medical issue if you find it's seemingly impossible to lose any weight. Your thyroid could be a possibility, or something else. That's common knowledge. It's best to check with your doctor, and it is also best to use the age-old advice of checking with your doctor before beginning any workout and nutritional plan as well. And remember, your gut area will probably be the last place you'll see any significant changes so don't fret if anything isn't happening there for a while. I've heard some interesting theories on this fact, though.

I remember hearing one crazy story about abdominal fat from an uninformed gym member at an old gym I use to go to regularly. It's pretty common to hear some pretty wacky stuff at the gym. I had a guy tell me and my gym partner Riff Johnson that his doctor told him he had a huge gut not because he had any fat in that area, but his waistline was bulging because there was so much muscle in his abdomen that it was pushing it outward. Yes, this is a true story, and it is also true that this is one of the most ridiculous excuses I've ever heard of for having a gut. This is as we know it, false; even if he did have huge ab muscles, it wouldn't make him look like he had a beer belly. Visceral fat is what causes this, and subcutaneous fat is what prevents you from seeing your abs muscles, so to achieve washboard six pack abs you have to burn off both kinds of fat. Visceral is the harder fat to get rid of, but keeping at it with diet and exercise will cause your abdominal area to shrink and expose those abs overtime.

In general, if you want to see your abs then you have to lower your body fat percentage, and the level you need to be at is different for men and women. The reason for this is women tend to carry more fat in other areas of the body than men, for example, women tend to carry more fat in the hip area probably due to the need for childbirth.[84] For men, if you can get your body fat down to ten-percent or below and women, thirteen-percent or below you should be starting to see your abs.[84] This is a generalized figure, remember each body is slightly different so exposing your abs is not an exact science; you may need to lower your body fat more or less depending on your genetics, and how muscular you are. The more muscular you are, the more your fat will be displaced to make room for the extra muscle.[85] It's also important to point out the fact that some people naturally carry more fat than others.[86] This is entirely up to your genes, but just because you may have more fat cells and naturally carry more fat than other body types doesn't mean you can't achieve the body of your dreams by proper diet, exercise routines and having a good healthy lifestyle.[86] It's my belief anyone has the possibility to get ripped, shredded, or whatever term you prefer.

Fat Loss, Weights vs. Cardio:

Contrary to popular belief, weight/strength training is effective in reducing body fat.[87] Cardio is not the end all be all activity for fat loss. When you lift weights, your metabolism stays jacked up for up to forty-eight hours after you are done with your workout, which means you continue to burn calories at a higher rate long after you are done lifting.[87] Part of the reason for this is the fact that your body has to work at repairing the microscopic tears you have caused from the all the lifting. It takes time to heal your muscles, and in that time your burning energy in the process. With cardio, you may burn more calories during the actual workout, but you're not going to get the same kind of "after burn" when you are finished with your workout.[87] Although cardio does tend to suppress appetite, and weight lifting does just the opposite. Either way, both kinds of exercise can have an effect on your body composition, and cause fat loss.

Be a Lifelong Fitness Learner:

The amount of knowledge we have about the human body and health and fitness, and how the body reacts to exercise and nutrition is light years ahead of where we were say a hundred years ago. However, knowledge is increasing at an alarming rate; new knowledge will likely be obtained in the future, new studies will be done, new theories tested, etc. The amount of knowledge will only increase, which is a good thing. The more science we learn and understand how fitness and nutrition act on our bodies, the more it could help us in reaching our health and fitness goals, and to get those ripped bodies we all want. Be a lifelong fitness learner. Theories are always changing, and it's important to know and study as much as you can, or want to if you have that sort of time if you can't hire a personal trainer.

Visualization is a Powerful Tool:

Out of everything that is an obstacle, or a helper in reaching your goals and obtaining your dreams, your mind is what controls where you end up more than anything else. More than your environment, influential people, and other factors, your mind can help you overcome amazingly difficult obstacles. If you want something bad enough you can figure out how to get it by using that powerful tool we have all been given.[88] If you want that perfect body, visualize in your mind exactly how you want to look. If you can create it in your mind, it can become your reality. Every idea, every man made thing in this world started in someone's mind. If you can realize the power behind that, there is nothing you can't achieve in the gym to get the body of your dreams, and there's nothing you can't achieve in life. Visualize it, and go to work.

New Year's Resolutions:

There is no one magical day of the year that if you start working towards your dreams or goals that you will have a better chance of success. We all know that probably more people make resolutions regarding going to the gym and getting in shape than any other kinds of New Year's resolutions. Waiting until New Year's Day to start working on your gym goals isn't going to make you more likely to succeed, and the keyword proving that is "waiting." If there were a magical day of the year to start working on your goals and dreams, it would be today! There is no reason to wait, stop making excuses and start working on those goals. You can make a resolution to do something right now, do not hesitate. Waiting for New Year's, or waiting until the start of the next week will not suddenly make you more committed. You have to fight through the pain of not wanting to do something you know you have to do in order to reach your goals.

I don't know how many times in the month of December I've heard people say that as soon as New

Year's hits their hitting the gym. Stop that, do it now, there is never a good time to start a major change, that's part of the reason why it's so hard to make changes, including putting yourself through the discomfort of working out hard because you want to look good come beach season. Decide on a course of action and don't hesitate. Great things don't happen to those who choose to wait; they happen for those who put the action in place and work for it. Action, rather than waiting can change your life for the better, and it can put you on the path towards your dream body.

All Workouts Are Not Created Equal:

Since no two bodies are exactly identical, it makes sense that not everyone's body is going to react the same way to any particular workout, or stimuli. This is an interesting fact, and it means you have to find out what your body responds to the best. For example, I've always had an easy time developing my pecs, but some chest exercises seem to have more of an effect on me than others, and vice versa for others. Also, I've discovered that with my strength training I always seem to see better and quicker results when I predominately use machines rather than free weights. However, I mix things up. I don't just use machines for strength/weight training, but I do prefer it, and it usually shows in the mirror.

The only way you're going to discover what your body prefers is through experience, and "feeling" it out. With experience and time you will naturally develop what I like to call brain-to-muscle instincts, and usually, your instincts are going to lead you to the right course of action. What I mean by this is hard to explain, but you can develop certain feelings, or a "taste" in what kind of exercises you want to do for different muscle groups on any given day. Brain-to- muscle instincts will only develop with a lot of experience, possibly years, but it's very helpful because your body will be telling you what it wants to do to adapt to the stresses you are putting on it.

Thirty Minutes of Hard Work Does Not Earn You A Day On the Couch:

Getting a hard workout in is a great accomplishment, and being consistent with your workouts is huge. However, what's best for your body is to have light to moderate physical activity throughout the day in addition to your workout. It's fantastic if you are consistently doing your workouts, but if you are sedentary for the remainder of the day, you will not see the best results. The human body was not meant to sit on a couch all day, or a desk. Unfortunately, if you have a sedentary job you may be at a disadvantage, but I would never advocate quitting your job as that would be foolish. In most cases, there are ways that you can incorporate some light to moderate activity in each and every day, even if you are forced to be sedentary for the better part of the day due to your job.

Think of different ways that you can get up and move around a bit. If you can, take stretch breaks at work as much as possible while still staying productive in your job. Go for a short walk on your breaks if that's a possibility. There are all kinds of ways you can squeeze in a little bit of movement here and there. When it comes time to be at home, just doing normal chores like taking out the trash or cleaning the house are a great and simple way to fill in the void in between your workouts. If you have kids, play with them (which you should be doing regardless). Although playing with your children may not seem like light activity at times, it's good for you and them, and it gives you an opportunity to spend some valuable time together. Take the dog for a walk, or go for a walk yourself - anything to get your body to do what it was meant to do, which is to move. If you have to go to the store, park the farthest away you can and use that as a little mini walk. Not including your workouts, small daily activities like these are much better than spending hours sitting on your couch or in front of your computer, or what have you. You don't have to spend all your time moving, but try to limit the amount of couch potato time, or inactivity as much as possible.

The opposite goes for those who have highly physical jobs. In cases like this, you can still do your workouts that will have a different kind of impact on your body's muscles and health, but you have to be very watchful of overtraining, and getting enough rest and sleep is crucial. Most physical blue collar jobs, as opposed to typically sedentary white collar jobs, do have a bit of an advantage when it comes to your bodies need for some form of physical activity throughout the day.

Finally, your job can keep you extremely busy and make it tough to find the time to move around let alone get a workout in. However, even in the most time challenging situations you can find the time to squeeze in what you know you must do to get the body of your dreams. You've got to want it bad enough, and if you do I assure you, there will be a way.

Remember Your "Why:"

Without a doubt, there will be days that motivation will seem non-existent. Occasional lack of motivation is normal, and I believe everyone goes through this at one point or another, and for one reason or another. Generally speaking, once you get moving, motivation will typically find you, but one way to find it at any time whether you're moving or not is to remember your "why." Only you can answer the question of "Why am I doing this? What is the purpose?" Always think back on this when you are having trouble staying motivated. No matter how trivial, or grand your reasoning may be for putting yourself through what some may view as the agony of a workout, let this be your number one driving factor. Whether it be something simple, such as wanting to look good when you hit the beach, or something big, like wanting to be a fitness model, to be healthier, to live longer to enjoy your grandkids, having more energy to play with your kids, to be a better athlete, or whatever reason it may be; your why will keep you pushing forward. Always maintain the end goal in mind, never lose focus of that.

Chapter Fifteen Summary:

- **FIIT: Frequency, intensity, time, and type of exercise. If you're not seeing results one of these factors must change, or a combination of factors, or all of them.**

- **Lack of intensity is the probably the number one reason why many never see results in the gym.**

- **Intensity techniques are great tools that can help you achieve the body of your dreams.**

- **Sleep is necessary for healing and change to take place in your body. Your body does the most muscle repair and building during sleep. Lack of sleep can mess with your hormones too.**

- If you're trying to build muscle, ZZZ's will get you inches. Do your best to get eight hours of sleep. If you're doing very intense workouts shoot for ten if you can.

- Although you can technically do cardio every day, you should take at least one day a week to completely rest.

- Take a small vacation (a week or so) from the gym occasionally. This will allow for full recovery.

- Only weigh yourself once a week. Don't obsess over the scale. Results are subtle, and best seen in the mirror.

- Weight fluctuation up or down within a few pounds is perfectly normal. Pay more attention to trends. Is your weight going down, up, or is it stable?

- Best time to step on the scale? In the a.m. after going to the bathroom and with little or no clothing on. The worst time to weigh yourself is at night.

- Keep in mind muscle gain and fat loss can occur at the same time resulting in little change in body weight. This is one reason why the mirror wins vs. the scale.

- The goal of weight loss is really fat loss. Muscle loss will slow your metabolism; an enemy of fat loss. More muscle equals a faster metabolism. Eat plenty of protein.

- Ignore ads that try to sell you on insanely fast fat loss products. Stick to the one to two pounds lost per week rule.

- When first experiencing weight loss, water, and glycogen (stored carbohydrates) will go first, then fat. Because of this, the first few weeks or so of weight loss can be higher than normal.

- You can't choose where you want to lose fat. Sit-ups won't automatically burn belly fat. It's entirely up to your genes where you shed fat first. Typically you will lose fat all over and the gut is the last to go because more fat is stored there, especially for men.

- Visceral fat is internal fat that is stored in the gut and around organs. This is the least healthy fat and causes belly bulge. Subcutaneous fat is what we see below the skin. Other internal fat is located in muscles, joints, etc.

- It's not uncommon to not see any results for at least six weeks when starting a workout regimen. This is because the body tends to hold onto water when suddenly placed under stress. If after six weeks there's still no results consult your doctor. You could have an underactive thyroid or another underlying medical condition.

- For men, body fat percentage below ten percent will typically result in a six-pack. For women, it's thirteen percent. This is a generalized figure, each body is different. The more muscle you have the more fat will be displaced, which will give you a more ripped look.

- Weight training can help you burn fat, not just cardio. Cardio burns more calories during the workout, but weights burn more after due to the fact your body has to heal the microscopic tears you just caused.

- Always stay up to date on current knowledge, which is increasing at an alarming rate.

- Your mind controls everything. Visualize the body of your dreams. If you can create it in your mind, it can become your reality.

- Never wait until New Year's, Monday, or tomorrow to start working on the body of your dreams. There is no magic day to get started that will increase your chances of success. Today is the day to start!

- **No two bodies will react the same to the same workout/stimuli. Discover what your body best responds to.**

- **After your workout don't just flop down on the couch for the rest of the day. You will not see the best results by doing this. Daily, light to moderate physical activity is what's best for your body.**

- **Sedentary jobs make physical activity throughout the day difficult, but be creative, look for ways to add in any kind of activity. For example, park further away in the parking lot to make you walk more.**

- **Remember your "why." The reason you are hitting the gym is your number one motivator, whether it's a big lofty goal or a small one.**

Final Thoughts:

My fitness journey from childhood to the present has been anything but glorious. In fact, it's been filled with countless frustrations ranging from nagging injuries, stale results, or to results, but then gut-wrenching setbacks, which have been mostly due to my own loss of motivation and willpower. It's been a continuous cycle, and in achieving the results I was seeking, maintaining those results has been just challenging as obtaining them in the first place. Because of all this I can say I've been in the trenches of wanting eye-popping results from my efforts in the gym, but not knowing how to achieve that seemingly impossible goal at times. Better yet, I've gone through the challenge of knowing what it takes to succeed in the gym, but then struggling with the application of that knowledge due to my own weaknesses. I've been at a point where most of you may have been, so I know how hard and frustrating it can be to see the changes you desire from all your hard work that you put into the gym. I've been overweight, lost the weight, and then gained it back again. I've been in superb shape and ripped before, and other times I've looked "soft." At times I've been hyper-focused and motivated, and other times I've dreaded having to pick up a dumbbell, or to do a dreaded burpee. I've been through all the emotions you can think of when it comes to trying to get in shape and look your best.

There have been times when I so badly did not want to do my workout that I would get into my own head and try to justify why I didn't need to work out that day. That's a battle, and battling with your own mind can be one of the toughest battles you can fight. Your mind can be your biggest asset or worst enemy. I can't tell you that achieving the body of your dreams will ever be at all easy because it won't be. It will be extremely challenging at times. I tell you this because it's a truth. Don't let that discourage you, though, because the harder the battle, the sweeter the victory. They say knowing is half the battle; well through intensive study, experience, and observation, I have been able to produce this product of knowledge, for you.

This book has been designed to circumvent the frustrations experienced by so many of us when we spend so much time trying to improve our bodies, only to feel like we are on a hamster wheel. First and foremost, everything starts in your mind. Your entire world is predominantly controlled by your mind. I am a passionate advocate for the power of positive thinking. I firmly believe that what you attract in your life is directly related to the kind of thinking you do, whether it be negative or positive. Be courageously confident that you can achieve what others have achieved before you. If you want a ripped body with six pack abs, you have to believe it's achievable, because it truly is. You have to unquestionably want it badly enough.

Generally, people get what they set out to achieve when they have an enormous amount of drive and willpower to go out and get it. The most successful people in the world share these same traits; extreme confidence, strong willpower, and an unbelievable drive to achieve what they set out to do. These traits carry over into any part of your life, whether it be in the gym, your home life, or professional life. All aspects of life are affected by these traits. And all these traits can be improved upon. Self-improvement has always been a strong interest of mine; something I believe can be worked on every single day. Believe in yourself, take the knowledge contained in this book and the results you can achieve with the application of this knowledge can be truly astounding. You can conquer mountains when you combine knowledge with action. Let this book be a guide, and a tool to teach you how to be fit smart. You will be so glad you did, and you will receive a natural boost in self-confidence, pride, and you'll be all the healthier and have a better quality of life for it. I believe that a healthy body can produce a happy mind, and happy minds can build a better world, and I think we'd all agree a more fit and happy world would be a pretty nice place to live in.

About the Author:
Marshall Nash

A Maine resident his whole life, Marshall Nash grew up in the small town of Pittsfield Maine. He spent much of his youth playing sports and learning the art of bodybuilding. He started weight lifting as a very young impressionable seven-year-old boy, and barring a few moments in life, has not put the weights down since. Sports and fitness have always been his number one passion, which subsequently drove him down a path to become a nationally certified personal fitness trainer for a number of years now in adulthood.

Through the years and many gym memberships, Marshall has collected a massive amount of knowledge on the subject of health and fitness. His mission is to share as much of that knowledge as possible with the world; and to educate as many as he can on not only what to do, but also on the avoidable mistakes that are made time and time again that hold individuals back from attaining their gym time goals. Marshall is a devoted father of two; daughter Kenzie and son Mikie. He has many interests that extend beyond health and fitness, one of them spending time with his children, family, and friends. A lover of people, Marshall continues to educate people through consultations and is in hopes of being an inspiration for what can be accomplished through willpower and dedication to one's goals in the gym, and in life.

One more thing:

Thank you for taking the time to read **Blunders In The Gym: Fitness Mistakes to Avoid for Physique Perfection.** If you enjoyed this book and found it to be useful for you I would be very grateful if you would post a review on Amazon. Your support and feedback is truly appreciated and it certainly does make a difference. I take the time to personally read all of the reviews so I can get your feedback and make this book the absolute best it can possibly be.

If you would like to leave a review for this book then you can simply visit the link below. Thank you so much for your support!

http://hyperurl.co/axeqmo

Other Books by Marshall A. Nash:

Blunders In The Kitchen: Diet Mistakes to Avoid
While Fueling the Perfect Beach Physique

Connect With Marshall A. Nash:

Thank you so much for taking the time to read this book. It is a blessing to be able to be your coach through this book. I'm excited for what the knowledge in this book can do for your health, and for what it can do to help you reach your goals and remain blunder free.

If you should have any questions of any kind feel free to contact me at: mailto:marshallnashauthor@gmail.com

You can follow me on Twitter: @MrMarshallNash

You can also connect with me on Facebook here: https://www.facebook.com/MarshallANash/

I'm wishing you the best of health, happiness, and success in reaching your goals!

Yours's In Health,

Marshall A. Nash

Notes

References:

1. Schwarzenegger, Arnold., and Dobbins, Bill. 1998. *The New Encyclopedia of Modern Bodybuilding*. Simon & Schuster. New York. "Mind in the Muscle." Pages 232-233.

2. Perez, Summer. 2017. "Mind-Body Connection To Maximize Your Workout." *Body Rock*. Accessed: December 23rd 2017. http://www.bodyrock.tv/fitness/mind-body-connection-maximize-workout/

3. Deane, Lisa. "Proper Training Gear and Also Footwear for Runners." Personal Fitness Trainer National Certification Course by World Instructor Training Schools from Kennebec Valley Community College, Fairfield, ME, April 21, 2012.

4. Casazza, Gerard. 2017. "Importance of Proper Form When Strength Training." *National Federation of Professional Trainers*. Accessed: December 23rd 2017. https://www.nfpt.com/blog/importance-proper-form-strength-training

5. Bushell, Dana. 2017. "Benefits of Proper Weight Lifting Technique." *Allmax*. Accessed: December 23rd 2017. http://www.allmaxnutrition.com/post-articles/training/benefits-of-proper-weight-lifting-technique/

6. Fetters, Aleisha K. 2016. "Why Range of Motion Matters for Your Strength Training Goals." *Daily Burn Life*. Accessed: December 23rd 2017. http://dailyburn.com/life/fitness/strength-training-range-of-motion/

7. Schwarzenegger, Arnold., and Dobbins, Bill. 1998. *The New Encyclopedia of Modern Bodybuilding*. Simon & Schuster. New York. "Range of Motion." Pages 140 and 397.

8. Deane, Lisa. "Sticking Points in Fitness Training." Personal Fitness Trainer National Certification Course by World Instructor Training Schools from Kennebec Valley Community College, Fairfield, ME, April 14, 2012.

9. Rdlfitness. 2017. "Sticking Points On Exercises." Accessed: December 23rd 2017. http://www.rdlfitness.com/sticking-points/

10. Deane, Lisa. "Proper Breathing during Exercise." Personal Fitness Trainer National Certification Course by World Instructor Training Schools from Kennebec Valley Community College, Fairfield, ME, March 31, 2012.

11. Smith, Stew. 2017. "Breathing During Exercise." *Military.com*. Accessed: December 23rd 2017. https://www.military.com/military-fitness/workouts/breathing-during-exercise

12. Deane, Lisa. "Eccentric and Concentric Movement." Personal Fitness Trainer National Certification Course by World Instructor Training Schools from Kennebec Valley Community College, Fairfield, ME, April 14, 2012.

13. Beardsley, Chris. 2017. "Why does eccentric training produce eccentric-specific strength gains? (strength is specific)." *The Strength & Conditioning Research Review*. Accessed: December 23rd 2017. https://www.strengthandconditioningresearch.com/perspectives/eccentric-training-different/

14. Mahler, Mike. 2015. "Workout Less & Achieve More." *Bodybuilding.com*. Accessed: December 23rd 2017. https://www.bodybuilding.com/fun/mahler62.htm

15. Mccahon, Jessica. 2017. "Reasons to Not Work the Same Muslces Every Day." *Livestrong.com*. Accessed: December 23rd 2017. https://www.livestrong.com/article/521047-reasons-to-not-work-the-same-muscles-every-day/

16. Hall, Brandon. 2015. "What Happens When You Do The Same Exercises Every Day?" *Stack Blue Star Sports*. Accessed: December 23rd 2017. http://www.stack.com/a/same-exercise-every-day

17. Deane, Lisa. "Cardio/Light Exercise Can Do Daily, but Recommend One Day of Rest." Personal Fitness Trainer National Certification Course by World Instructor Training Schools from Kennebec Valley Community College, Fairfield, ME, April 14, 2012.

18. Cheung, Hume, and Linda Maxwell. 2003. "Delayed Onset Muscle Soreness." *Trillium Fitness* page 145. Accessed: December 23rd 2017. http://www.trilliumfitness.co.uk/wp-content/uploads/2016/02/Chung-2003-DOMS.pdf

19. Deane, Lisa. "Abs, Calves, and Forearms Can Be Worked Every day." Personal Fitness Trainer National Certification Course by World Instructor Training Schools from Kennebec Valley Community College, Fairfield, ME, April 14, 2012.

20. Snyder, Zack, Kurt Johnstad, Michael B. Gordon, Frank Miller, Lynn Varley, and Mark Twight. 2006. "300: Special Features." Blu-Ray Disc. Directed by Zack Snyder. Warner Bros. Pictures.

21. Fetters, Aleisha K. 2014. "How to Achieve a Runner's High." *Runners World*. Accessed: December 23rd 2017. https://www.runnersworld.com/running-tips/how-to-achieve-a-runners-high

22. Vaillancourt, Joey. 2015. "7 Ways To Bust Any Plateau!" *Bodybuilding.com*. Accessed: December 23rd 2017. https://www.bodybuilding.com/fun/7-ways-to-bust-any-plateau.htm

23. Lanecc. 2013. "The Muscle Confusion Edition." *Lanecc.edu*. Accessed: January 7th 2018.https://www.lanecc.edu/sites/default/files/facilities/march182013 muscleconfusion.pdf

24. Deane, Lisa. "Habit Formation." Personal Fitness Trainer National Certification Course by World Instructor Training Schools from Kennebec Valley Community College, Fairfield, ME, April 21, 2012.

25. Howley T. Edward., Don Franks. 2007. *Fitness Professional's Handbook: Fifth Edition*. Human Kinetics. www.HumanKinetics.com. United States. "Overtraining Syndrom." Pages: 207-208.

26. Trotter, Kathleen. 2008. "Different Body Types React Differently to Exercise: Let me tell you why and how that happens." *Kathleen Trotter*. Accessed: December 23rd 2017. http://www.kathleentrotter.com/different-body-types-react-differently-to-exercise-let-me-tell-you-why-and-how-that-happens/

27. Schwarzenegger, Arnold., and Dobbins, Bill. 1998. *The New Encyclopedia of Modern Bodybuilding*. Simon & Schuster. New York. "Negative Reps." Page 190.

28. Suss, Jessica. 2017. "Here's Why Weight Loss Is 80 Percent Diet and 20 Percent Exercise." *Simple Most: make the most out of life*. Accessed: December 23rd 2017. https://www.simplemost.com/weight-loss-80-percent-diet-20-percent-exercise/

29. Deane, Lisa. "Better to Eat Five Small Meals a Day Than Three Big Ones." Personal Fitness Trainer National Certification Course by World Instructor Training Schools from Kennebec Valley Community College, Fairfield, ME, March 31, 2012.

30. Sepal, Jessica. 2013. "8 Ways To Balance Your Blood Sugar Naturally." *Mbgfood*. Accessed: December 26th 2017. https://www.mindbodygreen.com/0-10134/8-ways-to-balance-your-blood-sugar-naturally.html

31. Deane, Lisa. "Hierarchy of Digestible Foods." Personal Fitness Trainer National Certification Course by World Instructor Training Schools from Kennebec Valley Community College, Fairfield, ME, March 31, 2012.

32. Deane, Lisa. "Eat a Protein with Every Meal." Personal Fitness Trainer National Certification Course by World Instructor Training Schools from Kennebec Valley Community College, Fairfield, ME, March 31, 2012.

33. Schwarzenegger, Arnold., and Dobbins, Bill. 1998. *The New Encyclopedia of Modern Bodybuilding*. Simon & Schuster. New York. "Eat One Gram of Protein per Pound of Body Weight If You Want to Gain Muscle." Page 709.

34. Deane, Lisa. "Eat Half the Amount of Protein Grams as Body Weight When Trying to Lose Weight." Personal Fitness Trainer National Certification Course by World Instructor Training Schools from Kennebec Valley Community College, Fairfield, ME, March 31, 2012.

35. Deane, Lisa. "Fruit Juice Doesn't Have Fiber Content Like Eating Whole Fruit." Personal Fitness Trainer National Certification Course by World Instructor Training Schools from Kennebec Valley Community College, Fairfield, ME, March 31, 2012.

36. Hyman, Mark. 2016. "Sugar or Fat: What's Worse for Your Waistline?" *Cleveland Clinic*. Accessed: December 26th 2017. https://health.clevelandclinic.org/2016/02/sugar-vs-fat-which-is-worse-for-weight-gain/

37. Deane, Lisa. "Eating Whole Foods Is Better for You Than Processed Foods." Personal Fitness Trainer National Certification Course by World Instructor Training Schools from Kennebec Valley Community College, Fairfield, ME, March 31, 2012.

38. Whitman, Sarah. 2017. "Boiled Vegetables vs. Steamed." *Sfgate*. Accessed: December 26th 2017. http://healthyeating.sfgate.com/boiled-vegetables-vs-steamed-11028.html

39. Deane, Lisa. "Don't Eat or Workout Three Hours before Going to Bed." Personal Fitness Trainer National Certification Course by World Instructor Training Schools from Kennebec Valley Community College, Fairfield, ME, March 31, 2012.

40. Hutchins, Michael. 2017. "Does Exercise Raise Your Metabolic Rate for Several Hours After the Workout?" *Livestrong.com*. Accessed: December 26th 2017. https://www.livestrong.com/article/485498-does-exercise-raise-your-metabolic-rate-for-several-hours-after-the-workout/

41. Sfgate. 2017. "How to Know When Your Stomach Is Full & to Stop Eating?" *Sfgate*. Accessed: December 26th 2017. http://healthyeating.sfgate.com/stomach-full-stop-eating-3080.html

42. Google image. 2017. "Good Carbs vs Bad Carbs." Accessed: December 26th 2017. https://www.google.com/imgres?imgurl=https://foxvalleyfitness.files.wordpress.com/2015/02/good-carbs-vs-bad-carbs.jpg&imgrefurl=https://foxvalleyfitness.wordpress.com/2015/02/02/good-vs-bad-carbohydrates/&h=612&w=607&tbnid=bfdGDqVGi70EAM:&tbnh=160&tbnw=159&usg=___ndY7nHGUXVISCwVTXLyWKHPYfLE%3D&vet=1 0ahUKEwiG9I3Xh6nYAhVr6YMKHaZNAVEQ9QEILTAA..i&docid=XbJ 3ky2JajhskM&sa=X&ved=0ahUKEwiG9I3Xh6nYAhVr6YMKHaZNAVE Q9QEILTAA

43. Deane, Lisa. "Weight Training and Cardio Effect on Appetite." Personal Fitness Trainer National Certification Course by World Instructor Training Schools from Kennebec Valley Community College, Fairfield, ME, April 14, 2012.

44. Deane, Lisa. "How Much Water You Should Drink in a Day." Personal Fitness Trainer National Certification Course by World Instructor Training Schools from Kennebec Valley Community College, Fairfield, ME, March 31, 2012.

45. Howley T. Edward., Don Franks. 2007. *Fitness Professional's Handbook: Fifth Edition.* Human Kinetics. www.HumanKinetics.com. United States. "Every Chemical/Metabolic Process Requires Water." Page: 110.

46. Mayo Clinic. 2015. "Counting calories: Get back to weight-loss basics." Accessed: December 26th 2017. https://www.mayoclinic.org/healthy-lifestyle/weight-loss/in-depth/calories/art-20048065

47. Schwarzenegger, Arnold., and Dobbins, Bill. 1998. *The New Encyclopedia of Modern Bodybuilding.* Simon & Schuster. New York. "Don't Lose More Than Two Pounds of Fat per Week." Page 746.

48. Howley T. Edward., Don Franks. 2007. *Fitness Professional's Handbook: Fifth Edition.* Human Kinetics. www.HumanKinetics.com. United States. "Maintain a Food Journal." Pages: 110-112.

49. Deane, Lisa. "Starvation Eats Muscle and Slows Metabolism." Personal Fitness Trainer National Certification Course by World Instructor Training Schools from Kennebec Valley Community College, Fairfield, ME, March 31, 2012

50. Schwarzenegger, Arnold., and Dobbins, Bill. 1998. *The New Encyclopedia of Modern Bodybuilding.* Simon & Schuster. New York. "Too Much Rest Slows Your Heart Rate down and Less Muscle Fiber Engages". Page 148.

51. Deane, Lisa. "Different Muscle Fiber Types and Recovery Time for Each." Personal Fitness Trainer National Certification Course by World Instructor Training Schools from Kennebec Valley Community College, Fairfield, ME, March 24, 2012

52. Baggett, Kelly. 2007. "Understanding Muscle Fiber Types." *Bodybuilding.com.* Accessed: December 27th 2017. https://www.bodybuilding.com/fun/kelly13.htm

53. Deane, Lisa. "The Importance of Warming Up." Personal Fitness Trainer National Certification Course by World Instructor Training Schools from Kennebec Valley Community College, Fairfield, ME, March 31, 2012

54. Mealy, Clyde. 2017. "Why Is It Important to Cool down after Exercise?" *Sharecare.* Accessed: December 27th 2017.

https://www.sharecare.com/health/flexibility-training/why-important-cool-down-exercise

55. Deane, Lisa. "Warming up Prepares Body to Do Work and Can Prevent Injury." Personal Fitness Trainer National Certification Course by World Instructor Training Schools from Kennebec Valley Community College, Fairfield, ME, March 31, 2012.

56. Howley T. Edward., Don Franks. 2007. *Fitness Professional's Handbook: Fifth Edition*. Human Kinetics. www.HumanKinetics.com. United States. "The Importance of Warming up and Cooling Down." Page: 200.

57. Barlow, Rich. 2015. "Stretch Before Exercise? Not So Fast." *BU Today*. Accessed: December 27th 2017. https://www.bu.edu/today/2015/stretch-before-exercise-not-so-fast/

58. Daiwik. 2017. "What Is Ballistic Stretching Exercise And What Are Its Benefits?" *Stylecraze*. Accessed: December 27th 2017. http://www.stylecraze.com/articles/what-is-ballistic-stretching-exercise-and-benefits/#gref

59. Mind Tools. 2017. "Personal Goal Setting: Planning to Live Your Life Your Way." Accessed: December 27th 2017. https://www.mindtools.com/page6.html

60. Deane, Lisa. "Order of Exercises." Personal Fitness Trainer National Certification Course by World Instructor Training Schools from Kennebec Valley Community College, Fairfield, ME, April 14, 2012.

61. Mueller, Jen, and Nicole Nichols. 2008. "Reference Guide To Anaerobic Exercise: An In-Depth Look at High Intensity Exercise." *Spark People: Live Healthy & Happy*. Accessed: December 27th 2017. http://www.sparkpeople.com/resource/fitness_articles.asp?id=1035

62. Howley T. Edward., Don Franks. 2007. *Fitness Professional's Handbook: Fifth Edition*. Human Kinetics. www.HumanKinetics.com. United States. "Glycogen." Pages: 104.

63. Schwarzenegger, Arnold., and Dobbins, Bill. 1998. *The New Encyclopedia of Modern Bodybuilding*. Simon & Schuster. New York. "The Pump." Page: 68.

64. Deane, Lisa. "It Takes the Average Individual 20 Minutes of Exercise before You Dip into Fat Stores." Personal Fitness Trainer National Certification Course by World Instructor Training Schools from Kennebec Valley Community College, Fairfield, ME, March 24, 2012.

65. Deane, Lisa. "Work Your Larger Muscles First Smaller Second." Personal Fitness Trainer National Certification Course by World Instructor Training Schools from Kennebec Valley Community College, Fairfield, ME, April 14, 2012.

66. Baily, Joshua. 2017. "Big Vs. Small Muscles." *Livestron.com*. Accessed: December 27th 2017. https://www.livestrong.com/article/436440-big-vs-small-muscles/

67. Deane, Lisa. "FIIT." Personal Fitness Trainer National Certification Course by World Instructor Training Schools from Kennebec Valley Community College, Fairfield, ME, March 17, 2012.

68. Deane, Lisa. "Workouts Should Be at Least Ten Minutes Long for Any Real Benefits." Personal Fitness Trainer National Certification Course by World Instructor Training Schools from Kennebec Valley Community College, Fairfield, ME, April 14, 2012.

69. Kravits, Len. 2014. "High-Intensity Interval Training." *American College of Sports Medicine*. Accessed: December 30th 2017. https://www.acsm.org/docs/brochures/high-intensity-interval-training.pdf

70. LaMeaux, E.C. 2017. "What Is Steady State Cardio?" *Gaiam*. Accessed: December 30th 2017. https://www.gaiam.com/blogs/discover/what-is-steady-state-cardio

71. Bryant, Josh. 2016. "High-Intensity Interval Training: The Ultimate Guide." *Bodybuilding.com*. Accessed: December 30th 2017. https://www.bodybuilding.com/content/high-intensity-interval-training-the-ultimate-guide.html

72. Schwarzenegger, Arnold., and Dobbins, Bill. 1998. *The New Encyclopedia of Modern Bodybuilding*. Simon & Schuster. New York. "Intensity Techniques." Pages: 187-198.

73. Deane, Lisa. "Sleep Is When Healing, Building Muscle, and Strength Occurs." Personal Fitness Trainer National Certification Course by World Instructor Training Schools from Kennebec Valley Community College, Fairfield, ME, April 14, 2012.

74. Bergland, Christopher. 2013. "Insomnia Increases Junk Food Cravings." *Psychology Today*. Accessed: December 30th 2017. https://www.psychologytoday.com/blog/the-athletes-way/201308/insomnia-increases-junk-food-cravings

75. Mann, Denise. 2017. "Sleep and Weight Gain." *WebMD*. Accessed: December 30th 2017. https://www.webmd.com/sleep-disorders/features/lack-of-sleep-weight-gain#1

76. Smith, Jessica. 2017. "When Your Weight Fluctuates: What's Normal and What's Not?" *Shape*. Accessed: December 30th, 2017.

77. Deane, Lisa. "It's Not Abnormal to Lose Some Muscle When Losing Weight, but Resistance Training and Eating Enough Protein Can Help Keep This to a Minimum." Personal Fitness Trainer National Certification Course by World Instructor Training Schools from Kennebec Valley Community College, Fairfield, ME, April 14, 2012.

78. Deane, Lisa. "Body Will Use up Glycogen before Fat When Working out to Lose Weight." Personal Fitness Trainer National Certification Course by World Instructor Training Schools from Kennebec Valley Community College, Fairfield, ME, March 31, 2012.

79. Howley T. Edward., Don Franks. 2007. *Fitness Professional's Handbook: Fifth Edition.* Human Kinetics. www.HumanKinetics.com. United States. "You Can't Spot Reduce Fat - Fat Loss Occurs All over the Body." Pages: 185.

80. Deane, Lisa. "Fat Loss Occurs All over Body According to Genetics." Personal Fitness Trainer National Certification Course by World Instructor Training Schools from Kennebec Valley Community College, Fairfield, ME, March 24, 2012.

81. Doheny, Kathleen. 2017. "The Truth A bout Fat." *WebMD*. Accessed: December 30th 2017. https://www.webmd.com/diet/features/the-truth-about-fat#1

82. Deane, Lisa. "Locations and Kinds of Body Fat." Personal Fitness Trainer National Certification Course by World Instructor Training Schools from Kennebec Valley Community College, Fairfield, ME, March 31, 2012.

83. Blokker, Shaun. 2013. "Having a Hard Time Losing Weight with INSANITY?"Youtube vide, 3:58. Published March 17th, 2013. Accessed: January 8th, 2018. https://www.youtube.com/watch?v=DNdCGW5fJ44

84. Deane, Lisa. "Body Fat Distribution for Men and Women and Percentages for Visible Abs." Personal Fitness Trainer National Certification Course by World Instructor Training Schools from Kennebec Valley Community College, Fairfield, ME, March 31, 2012.

85. Deane, Lisa. "Muscle Displaces Fat." Personal Fitness Trainer National Certification Course by World Instructor Training Schools from Kennebec Valley Community College, Fairfield, ME, April 14, 2012.

86. Schwarzenegger, Arnold., and Dobbins, Bill. 1998. *The New Encyclopedia of Modern Bodybuilding*. Simon & Schuster. New York. "Body Types/Some Naturally Have More Fat Cells." Page: 162.

87. Deane, Lisa. "You Can Lose Weight Lifting Weights/"after Burn" Due to Weight Lifting Can Raise Metabolism for up to 48 Hours Due to the Healing Process for Microscopic Muscle Fiber Tears." Personal Fitness Trainer National Certification Course by World Instructor Training Schools from Kennebec Valley Community College, Fairfield, ME, April 14, 2012.

88. Canfield, Jack. 2017. "Visualization Techniques to Affirm Your Desired Outcomes: A Step-by-Step Guide." *JackCanfield.com*. Accessed: December 30th 2017. http://jackcanfield.com/blog/visualize-and-affirm-your-desired-outcomes-a-step-by-step-guide/